MOLECULAR INSIGHT OF DRUG DESIGN

Edited by **Arli Aditya Parikesit**

Molecular Insight of Drug Design
http://dx.doi.org/10.5772/intechopen.71744
Edited by Arli Aditya Parikesit

Contributors

Kaori Nomura, Brian Edwords, Francisco Torrens, Gloria Castellano, Seema Kohli, Gul Shahnaz, Maria Hassan Kiani, Masoom Yasinzai, Lionel Gamarra, Debora Vieira, Arli Aditya Parikesit

First published in London, United Kingdom, 2018 by IntechOpen
IntechOpen is the global imprint of INTECHOPEN LIMITED, registered in England and Wales, registration number: 11086078, The Shard, 25th floor, 32 London Bridge Street
London, SE19SG – United Kingdom
Printed in Croatia

British Library Cataloguing-in-Publication Data
A catalogue record for this book is available from the British Library

Additional hard copies can be obtained from orders@intechopen.com

Molecular Insight of Drug Design, Edited by Arli Aditya Parikesit
p. cm.
Print ISBN 978-1-78923-632-3
Online ISBN 978-1-78923-633-0

For EU product safety concerns:
IN TECH d.o.o., Prolaz Marije Krucifikse Kozulić 3, 51000 Rijeka, Croatia,
info@intechopen.com or visit our website at intechopen.com.

Meet the editor

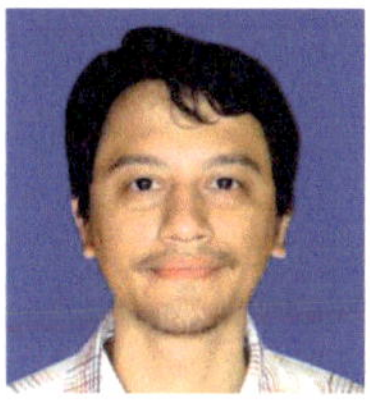

Arli Aditya Parikesit is the Head of Bioinformatics Department of School of Life Sciences, Indonesia International Institute for Life Sciences. He finished his bachelor and master from Department of Chemistry, Faculty of Mathematics and Sciences, University of Indonesia, and his Ph.D. from Faculty of Mathematics and Informatics, University of Leipzig, Germany with the support of DAAD fellowship of the German government. He has written more than 30 scientific publications on bioinformatics and has expertise in structural bioinformatics, and genome annotation methods.

Contents

Preface

The studies o drug design have improved significantly over this decade, starting with the implementation of nimotuzumab as a chemotherapy agent for glioma and squamous cell carcinomas. In this respect, nimotuzumab was design by taking into consideration the advances in molecular biology, especially in proteomics study, with blocking the Epidermal Growth Factor Receptor (EGFR). Some approaches, whether it is computationally-based, or wet experimentally-based, has made the improvement of nimotuzumab into a much safer chemotherapy agent. In this end, science has seen some interesting progress that possibly could follow the successful example of nimotuzumab. The multidisciplinary nature of drug design has opened many new possibilities in combating pathogens or other cause for diseases. Although the role of medical, pharmacy, and nursery studies still be a focal point for drug design, the rising roles of the multidisciplinary sciences are taking place as well.

The approaches in drug design are mainly comprised of these three multidisciplinary sciences. First, Bioinformatics has successfully gather biological data in form of biomolecular sequences, in order to construct knowledge on drug and vaccine design. It is of considerable importance for drug designers to comprehend the utilization of bioinformatics tools for resolving their research questions. Second, Nanotechnology has made possible the design and delivery of the nano-based drug. Third, Pharmaceutical Chemistry made it possible to investigate the adsorption, distribution, metabolism, and toxicology of the drug candidates in a fine-grained resolution. Although other approaches could be in place, the three of them are noted for providing a significant contribution to drug design. It is noticeable that many research groups have consisted of multidisciplinary team members with at least professionals in those three approaches. As drug design is becoming needier in experts in those approaches, study programs in bioinformatics, nanotechnology, and pharmaceutical chemistry are enacted to educate and trains experts in those particular fields. Those programs are enacted as early as Bachelor level because the multidisciplinary approaches should be emphasized as early as possible. The program managers of those study programs could be from diverse backgrounds, whether they are medical doctors, biologist, chemist, physicist, informaticians, engineers or others, but they should act as the scientist that love to work in a multidisciplinary environment and willing to defend the interest of many different scientific approaches accordingly. In this end, the graduates of those study programs are working together in a very diverse background team for constructing novel design of modern drugs. This book is indeed showing that such initiatives are in place at academia and industry. In this end, it could be stated that the goal of this book is to give the clear picture of how those different approaches worked in solving problems in drug design.

Hopefully, this book will be a significant contribution to the resolution of the world's health problems in relation to the complexity of drug design. This contribution will be useful to students, researcher, industrialist, and even the business development of drug companies, in order to anticipate the future menace of human health. It could be seen that after the elucidation of modern molecular-based medication, the human health problems are still there. The cure for cancer is still yet on the way, while some diseases such as Tuberculosis are re-emerged as antibiotic-resistant strain. Multidisciplinary approaches could be promising in resolving those issues because they observed scientific phenomenon based upon a very diverse perspective that could enrich each other into much more holistic problem-solving pieces of advice.

Thus, in order to facilitate easy reading, this book is divided into two sections. The first section will discuss General Information and Quality Control in Drug Design. This particular section will primarily emphasize on the general features of modern drug design and how to ensure its fine-grained quality control for consistent production outlook. It comprises of three chapters. The Chapter 1, introductory chapter will be useful for explaining the current trend in drug design.will discuss. The Chapter 2 will discuss Framework of Evaluating Qualitative and Quantitative Information on Drug Safety. Lastly, the chapter 3 will discuss Integrated Approach to Nature as Source of New Drug Lead.

While the second section will discuss Specific Molecular Mechanism and Lead Compounds for Drug Design. This particular section will primarily emphasize on the biomolecular and biochemical mechanism of drugs in a cell or in the laboratory. It comprises of four chapters. The Chapter 4 will discuss Molecular Classification of anti-tubulin Agents with Indole Ring Binding at Colchicine Binding site. The Chapter 5 will discuss Multifunctional Polymeric Enveloped Nanocarriers: Targeting Extracellular and Intracellular Barriers. The Chapter 6 will discuss Multifunctional Nanoparticles for Successful Targeted Drug Delivery and Diagnostics Across Blood-Brain Barrier. gnostics Across Blood-Brain Barrier.

Based on those particular studies as aforementioned before, the future of drug design will be, fortunately, moving towards a much more multidisciplinary nature. Moreover, the current state of higher education and industry is on a very good moment in order to align themselves with this current development in drug design.

Arli Aditya Parikesit
Head of Bioinformatics Department
School of Life Sciences
Indonesia International Institute for Life Sciences
Indonesia

Section 1

General Information and Quality Control in Drug Design

Chapter 1

Introductory Chapter: The Contribution of Bioinformatics as Blueprint Lead for Drug Design

Arli Aditya Parikesit

Additional information is available at the end of the chapter

http://dx.doi.org/10.5772/intechopen.79664

1. Bioinformatics and drug design

Drugs are the most utilized pharmacobiochemicals for sustaining human's health. Previously, the drug was designed unintentionally and mostly with trial and error. The well-known example is the discovery of antibiotics by Alexander Fleming which was found unintentionally [1]. However, as pharmaceutical technology is gaining momentum with the advance of molecular biology, the genome technology was applied as well to assist the development of the novel drugs. It has given a way for the development of the new kind of science, bioinformatics, which is a multidisciplinary study to integrate molecular biology and information technology [2]. There are some methods in bioinformatics that provided assistance to drug design. They are, namely, sequence alignment for determining the conservation of genome and proteome; homology modeling for determining the protein model; molecular docking method to enable high-performance screening of large amounts of lead compound [3]; molecular dynamics to set the standard to comprehend the trajectory of lead compound, as well as its interaction [4]; and ADME-TOX method to enable fine-grained detection of pharmacological and toxicological properties of lead compounds [5]. Those methods are eventually used as blueprint lead for molecular cloning or genetic engineering experiment to generate high throughput molecular profiling of the drug leads, as a means of rational drug design approach [6].

2. Rational design of drugs

The implementations of rational drug design made it possible to customize drugs at the molecular and structural level. The possibilities are enormous as the molecular design is only limited by the extent of the available computational power. The availability of commercial cyclic peptide database has made possible to design drugs in various molecular configurations of peptide sequences [7, 8]. However, the classical approach of the isolation of natural product-based is still in use due to the availability of its respective database [9]. Moreover, due to the influence of natural product chemistry, the design of semisynthetic or synthetic-based compounds is still on demands [10]. Researchers also look for a smarter pathway to deliver drug such as utilizing E-cadherin-based drug design [11].

Although the rational drug design approach has provided groundbreaking innovations such as the development of antiretroviral/HIV drugs and smart anticancer chemotherapy agent such as nimotuzumab, it does not mean that the progression of life-threatening diseases has been halted [12, 13]. The complexity of disease's molecular mechanism has long baffled the biomedical researchers. The threat of multidrug antibiotic resistance bugs, pandemic viral infections (Ebola, avian influenza, MERS-CO, etc.), and civilization disease such as aging is pushing the researchers to develop much more advanced drug designs. In this end, the intelligence modifications of existing bioinformatics methods are devised to propose the novel way of developing drugs. The fragment-based docking method was utilized in order to construct drugs based upon the molecular fragment database [14]. Moreover, the reverse docking method was devised to optimize the lead compounds based on the proteomics library [15–17]. Finally, the development of transcriptomics approach enables researchers to develop the new breed of drugs, such as silencing(si)RNA-based lead compounds [18]. In this end, the smart design enables novel wet laboratory experimental methods such as the blood-brain barrier drug design method [19] and high throughput screening [20]. Thus, the molecular elucidation of the drug could be elucidated in a fine-grained manner using the NMR and crystallography instruments that are already commonly utilized in the field of protein crystallography [21]. Based on the advanced crystallography techniques, more proteins structure is already elucidated. This could be a great help in providing fine-grained receptor structures for rational drug design. Moreover, although crystallizing RNA molecules are tougher than protein, more RNA structures are already elucidated and deposited in the online database [22].

3. Outlook

As bioinformatics and protein crystallography are getting their momentum to contribute greatly in the study of rational drug design, it is found that the molecular mechanism of diseases is possible should be revealed based upon post genomics and proteomics approaches especially transcriptomics and epigenetics-based ones. The interplay of transcriptomics and epigenetics in the molecular mechanism of disease should be considered as primary information in the biomedical research [23]. Moreover, due to the influx of transcriptomics data, RNA structure elucidation is getting a momentum to be considered as a blueprint in drug design [24]. In this end, due to the specificity of the human genetic fingerprint, personalized medicine was developed where each patient got different medication depending on their genomics fingerprint [25–27]. The role of big data and artificial intelligence methods will be crucial in screening the influx of omics data in order to generate useful information to be revealed as the blueprint of drug design.

Author details

Arli Aditya Parikesit

Address all correspondence to: johnkecops@gmail.com

Head of Bioinformatics Department, School of Life Sciences, Indonesia International Institute for Life Sciences, Indonesia

References

[1] Kingston W. Antibiotics, invention and innovation. Research Policy. 2000;**29**:679-710. Available from: http://www.sciencedirect.com/science/article/pii/S0048733399000451 [Accessed: Nov 12, 2013]

[2] Hagen JB. The origins of bioinformatics. Nature Reviews. Genetics. 2000;**1**:231-236. DOI: 10.1038/35042090

[3] Shoichet BK, McGovern SL, Wei B, Irwin JJ. Lead discovery using molecular docking. Current Opinion in Chemical Biology. 2002;**6**:439-446. DOI: 10.1016/S1367-5931(02)00339-3

[4] Karplus M, McCammon JA. Molecular dynamics simulations of biomolecules. Nature Structural Biology. 2002;**35**:646-652. Available from: http://www.ncbi.nlm.nih.gov/pubmed/12198485

[5] van de Waterbeemd H, Gifford E. ADMET in silico modelling: Towards prediction paradise?, Nature Reviews. Drug Discovery. 2003;**2**:192-204. DOI: 10.1038/nrd1032

[6] Lionta E, Spyrou G, Vassilatis DK, Cournia Z. Structure-based virtual screening for drug discovery: Principles, applications and recent advances. Current Topics in Medicinal Chemistry. 2014;**14**:1923-1938. DOI: 10.2174/1568026614666140929124445

[7] Tambunan USF, Alkaff AH, Nasution MAF, Parikesit AA, Kerami D. Screening of commercial cyclic peptide conjugated to HIV-1 Tat peptide as inhibitor of N-terminal heptad repeat glycoprotein-2 ectodomain Ebola virus through in silico analysis. Journal of Molecular Graphics & Modelling. 2017;**74**:366-378. DOI: 10.1016/j.jmgm.2017.04.001

[8] Parikesit AA, Kinanty USFT. Screening of commercial cyclic peptides as inhibitor envelope protein dengue virus (DENV) through molecular docking and molecular dynamics. Pakistan Journal of Biological Sciences. 2013;**16**:1836-1848. DOI: 10.3923/pjbs.2013.1836.1848

[9] Tambunan USF, Parikesit A, Nasution MAF, Hapsari A, Kerami D. Exposing the molecular screening method of Indonesian natural products derivate as drug candidates for cervical cancer (summer 2017). Iranian Journal of Pharmaceutical Research. 2017;**16**:1113-1127. Available form: http://ijpr.sbmu.ac.ir/article_2088.html

[10] Tambunan USF, Parikesit AA, Ghifari AS, Satriyanto CP. In silico identification of 2-oxo-1,3-thiazolidine derivatives as novel inhibitors candidate of class II histone deacetylase

(HDAC) in cervical cancer treatment. Arabian Journal of Chemistry. 2015;**1**:1-6. DOI: 10.1016/j.arabjc.2015.07.010

[11] Prasasty VD, Tambunan USF, Siahaan TJ. Homology modeling and molecular dynamics studies of EC1 domain of VE-cadherin to elucidate docking interaction with cadherin-derived peptide. OnLine Journal of Biological Sciences. 2014;**14**:155. DOI: 10.3844/ojbsci.2014.155.162

[12] Lengauer T, Sing T. Bioinformatics-assisted anti-HIV therapy. Nature Reviews. Microbiology. 2006;**4**:790-797. DOI: 10.1038/nrmicro1477

[13] Spicer J. Technology evaluation: Nimotuzumab, the Center of Molecular Immunology/YM BioSciences/Oncoscience. Current Opinion in Molecular Therapeutics. 2005;**7**:182-191. Available from: http://www.ncbi.nlm.nih.gov/pubmed/15844627 [Accessed: May 4, 2018]

[14] Chen Y, Shoichet BK. Molecular docking and ligand specificity in fragment-based inhibitor discovery. Nature Chemical Biology. 2009;**5**:358-364. DOI: 10.1038/nchembio.155

[15] Lee A, Lee K, Kim D. Using reverse docking for target identification and its applications for drug discovery. Expert Opinion on Drug Discovery. 2016;**11**:707-715. DOI: 10.1080/17460441.2016.1190706

[16] Lee M, Kim D. Large-scale reverse docking profiles and their applications, BMC Bioinformatics. 2012;**13**(Suppl 1):S6. DOI: 10.1186/1471-2105-13-s17-s6

[17] Kharkar PS, Warrier S, Gaud RS. Reverse docking: A powerful tool for drug repositioning and drug rescue. Future Medicinal Chemistry. 2014;**6**:333-342. DOI: 10.4155/fmc.13.207

[18] Tafer H, Ameres SL, Obernosterer G, Gebeshuber CA, Schroeder R, Martinez J, Hofacker IL. The impact of target site accessibility on the design of effective siRNAs. Nature Biotechnology. 2008;**26**:578-583. DOI: 10.1038/nbt1404

[19] Prasasty VD, Krause ME, Tambunan USF, Anbanandam A, Laurence JS, Siahaan TJ. 1H, 13C and 15N backbone assignment of the EC-1 domain of human E-cadherin. Biomolecular NMR Assignments. 2015;**9**:31-35. DOI: 10.1007/s12104-013-9539-6

[20] Blondelle SE, Lohner K. Optimization and high-throughput screening of antimicrobial peptides. Current Pharmaceutical Design. 2010;**16**:3204-3211. Available form: http://www.ncbi.nlm.nih.gov/pubmed/20687884 [Accessed: Mar 8, 2013]

[21] Ferreon JC, Volk DE, Luxon BA, Gorenstein DG, Hilser VJ. Solution structure, dynamics, and thermodynamics of the native state ensemble of the Sem-5 C-terminal SH3 domain. Biochemistry. 2003;**42**:5582-5591. DOI: 10.1021/bi030005j

[22] Coimbatore Narayanan B, Westbrook J, Ghosh S, Petrov AI, Sweeney B, Zirbel CL, Leontis NB, Berman HM. The nucleic acid database: New features and capabilities. Nucleic Acids Research. 2014;**42**:D114-D122. DOI: 10.1093/nar/gkt980

[23] Fachrul M, Utomo DH, Parikesit AA. lncRNA-based study of epigenetic regulations in diabetic peripheral neuropathy. Silico Pharmacology. 2018;**6**:7. DOI: 10.1007/s40203-018-0042-8

[24] Parikesit AA, Utomo DH, Karimah N. Determination of secondary and tertiary structures of cervical cancer lncRNA diagnostic and siRNA therapeutic biomarkers. Indian Journal of Biotechnology. 2018;**23**:1. DOI: 10.22146/ijbiotech.28508

[25] Youngblood MW, Erson-Omay EZ, Günel M. Personalized medicine through advanced genomics. In: Malig. Brain Tumors. Cham: Springer International Publishing; 2017. pp. 31-48. DOI: 10.1007/978-3-319-49864-5_3

[26] Pi C, Zhang M, Peng X, Zhang Y, Xu C, Zhou Q. Liquid biopsy in non-small cell lung cancer: A key role in the future of personalized medicine? Expert Review of Molecular Diagnostics. 2017;**17**:1089-1096. DOI: 10.1080/14737159.2017.1395701

[27] Tsimberidou A-M. Initiative for molecular profiling and advanced cancer therapy and challenges in the implementation of precision medicine. Current Problems in Cancer. 2017;**41**:176-181. DOI: 10.1016/j.currproblcancer.2017.02.002

Chapter 2

Frameworks for Evaluating Qualitative and Quantitative Information on Adverse Drug Events throughout Development through to Marketing

Kaori Nomura and Brian David Edwards

Additional information is available at the end of the chapter

http://dx.doi.org/10.5772/intechopen.76331

Abstract

Significant public health issues caused by adverse drug reactions in the post-marketing phase, such as birth defects by thalidomide, have been well described. Unfortunately, subjects in clinical trials cannot completely avoid severe harm during drug development. TGN1412 in 2006 and BIA 10-2474 in 2016 were withdrawn from development due to severe adverse reactions in first-into-man studies. Thus, monitoring drug safety is important throughout all phases of development. In twenty-first century, minimizing drug development cost and time is a challenge for pharmaceutical companies. When a drug is approved with a smaller size and fewer number of clinical trials, pharmacovigilance and benefit-risk evaluation after marketing need to be sufficiently performed. Underpinned by understanding of the traditional methods of evaluating adverse drug reactions, new developments in IT and computing might well help us to detect drug safety signals earlier, enabling prompt intervention for protecting the rights of subjects and public health.

Keywords: risk management, pharmacovigilance, DSUR, PSUR, ADR, causality

1. Introduction

A new drug application dossier, accompanied with the Common Technical Document (CTD), needs to provide a risk management plan, and a marketing authorization holder needs to set up both the policy framework and a quality system for pharmacovigilance. This approach has become more important and valuable in regulating drugs, because the novelty, rarity, or technical specificity of drugs produces complexities to evaluating efficacy and safety.

Furthermore, in this decade, the risk-based approach for application has been proposed to address and evaluate potential risks associated with the clinical use of medicines, with regard to quality, safety, and efficacy. While the risk-based approach is to be differentiated from the risk management system or the benefit-risk assessment for evaluating marketing authorization, the idea is very close to it. This chapter introduces pharmacovigilance in the clinical development phase, especially with the aim of stimulating discussion about identification of risks associated with the clinical use of drugs qualitatively and quantitatively.

1.1. What to do when any clinical safety problem happen in the development phase?

Throughout the history, humans have used a variety of different therapies to treat injuries and diseases. During the nineteenth century, medicines were developed by separating, isolating, and extracting certain active ingredients from medicinal plants, e.g., morphine, quinine, and ephedrine. Then, in twentieth century, chemists discovered new chemicals, e.g., penicillin and streptomycin, from bacteria and synthesized better chemical substances of sulfonamides. In the first decades of twenty-first century, the development of drugs had been dramatically changed. Pharmaceuticals benefit from advances in all fields relating to medicine, e.g. pharmacology, physiology, and biochemistry, and were derived from synthetic compounds to target a certain site of action. For example, the progresses in medical science helped to reveal many of the mechanisms of the pathophysiological and pharmacological effects at the molecular level; for example, cimetidine and histamine-2 receptor blocker, which was a break through pharmacotherapy at that time for gastric ulcer. Molecular-targeted drugs now have been developed to treat various diseases, especially targeting specifically expressed molecules of cancer cells, e.g., imatinib.

Common to all pharmaceuticals is that they can bring both benefits and risks to humans. Thalidomide, which is now administered with dexamethasone to multiple myeloma patients, used to be first sold in West Germany as a sedative or hypnotic drug in 1950s, and then it was withdrawn from the market in 1961, because it was found to be responsible for teratogenic deformities in children based on reports of children of those mothers who took thalidomide during pregnancy. This tragedy was both a pre- and post-marketing landmark; countries recognized the need of adequate testing of medicines prior to marketing, the regulation of medicines, and the systems to identify the adverse effects of medicines as well as the potential relationship between marketing claims and safety [1, 2]. Because of the need for effective therapies in myeloma, thalidomide demonstrated sufficient benefit to achieve authorization and turned around the balance of benefit-risk from negative evaluation. This depended on effective risk minimization to prevent pregnancies in those who receive thalidomide.

International activities actively promoted regulations and empirical knowledge on clinical development in 1990s. However, in twenty-first century, one programme of an investigational medicinal product was withdrawn due to serious adverse reactions in the first-in-human clinical trial in 2006. This was known as TGN1412, a CD28 superagonist monoclonal antibody. Six volunteers were seriously afflicted by a cytokine-release syndrome requiring intensive care just after they received a bolus injection of TGN1412.

Although many new drugs implement a lifecycle risk management, another tragedy in clinical trial happened with a dose-finding study for BIA 10-2474, an experimental fatty acid amide hydrolase inhibitor for the treatment of anxiety disorder, Parkinson's disease, etc. An acute and rapid progressive neurologic syndrome developed on the fifth day of BIA 10-2474 administration (50 mg). The underlying mechanism of adverse drug reaction is still unknown regarding BIA 10-274, but it is supposed to be associated with drug accumulation as no clinical severe adverse events had been observed in single dose (0.25–100 mg) and 10-day administration (0.25–20 mg) [3].

The stories addressed above are extreme examples. However, a number of drug development programmes have been abandoned because of safety concerns or lack of efficacy. As mentioned in ICH Good Clinical Practice (GCP) [4], "A trial should be initiated and continued only if the anticipated benefit justifies the risks." Thus, sponsors need to make sure that benefit for patients should overweigh risk to patients. Information sharing and a system for risk management throughout the lifecycle of drugs from preclinical, clinical, and post-marketing are crucial, and this is reflected in the development safety update report (DSUR) which had been proposed [5] and then taken forward by the International Conference on Harmonization of Technical Requirements for Registration of Pharmaceuticals for Human Use (ICH) [6]. This emphasizes the importance of the principle of the benefit-risk balance, which is supported by pharmacovigilance concepts which originally emerged in the post-marketing phase.

1.2. The latest strategy to promote marketing a new medicine

Drugs are approved based on the evidence of efficacy and acceptable level of harm that have been observed during clinical trials. Now, to tackle remaining unmet needs of patients globally, the regulatory schemes for supporting early access have been adopted, such as compassionate use, accelerated assessment by regulatory agencies, and conditional marketing authorization. If it is expected to have new medicines with conditional use, an applicant is allowed to provide comprehensive data after approval. Once such a new medicine is approved, definitely, there is little evidence of efficacy and safety in real-world practice, so that effective pharmacovigilance should produce the important data to supplement the evidence as well as cost savings for an applicant in the drug development. As we receive more applications of early access program, the more careful that we should be to pay attention with not to confusing "absence of evidence" with "evidence of absence" at approval. It is critical to detect precisely and promptly the harms potentially caused by an investigated drug (monitoring), to assess individual cases (qualitative evaluation) and comparative groups as planned (quantitative evaluation), and to finalize benefit-risk assessment at defined points in time (**Figure 1**).

How we can define "risk" then? According to the International Organization for Standardization, risk is the "effect of uncertainty on objectives" [7] and in terms of drug development, the objectives are patients' and public health. Another definition can be "combination of the probability of occurrence of harm and the severity of that harm" for medical devices and manufacturing medicinal products [8, 9]. As such, risks related to use of a drug is defined "any risk relating to the quality, safety or efficacy of the medicinal product as regards patients' health

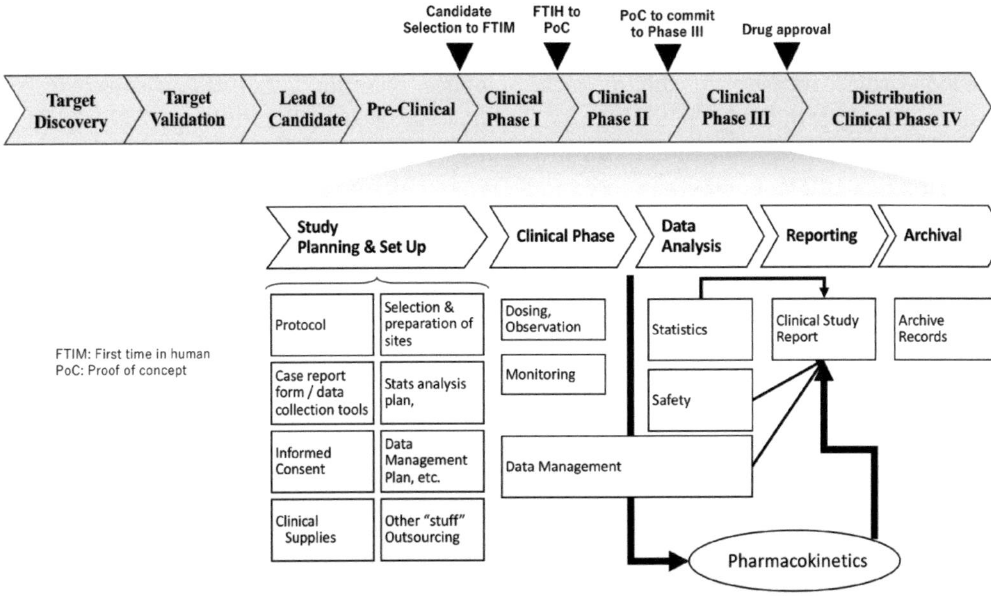

Figure 1. Drug development process and clinical data review. The figure is arranged and restructured from some of slides provided with the kind permission of the Product Safety Culture Initiative in the Alliance for Clinical Research Excellence and Safety.

or public health and any risk of undesirable effects on the environment" [10]. In traditional pharmacovigilance, the concept of risk concerns adverse drug reactions [11], as described later, however EU regulations now emphasize that it is as been expanded to include ineffective use outside the label, misuse and abuse. In reality for pharmacovigilance, we propose to bear in mind other systematic factors impacting risks of medicines as well (such as facilities, procedures, computerized systems) that may cause medication errors. Those risks cannot be evaluated enough in drug development, therefore the plan is necessary to continue vigilance once marketed and take action once a potential harm is identified. Thus pharmacovigilance has become even more important to manage various safety problems with these new rapid access regulatory approvals.

Risk management encompasses "risk assessment" and "risk minimization" with the management cycle to assess, implement, evaluate, and modify safety measures; the former is to identify and characterize the nature, frequency, and severity of the risks associated with the use of a product, as focused in this chapter; the latter is to minimize or mitigate a product's risks through communication, education, and restriction of use while preserving its benefit.

2. Pharmacovigilance in clinical trials

Data obtained from clinical trials vary depending on the situation of an investigational substance and those are different from post-marketing data; the patient being administered can be perfectly observed, the number of patients is small, and the information on subjects can be biased under restrictions of subjects' health background. As with post-marketing data collection, the data collection method is an essential element of the pharmacovigilance process during clinical trial with proper data collection to enable analysis of medical interpretation of the case narrative and the aggregated data. Evaluation of case information obtained in clinical trials is possible by use of the approaches cultivated in pharmacovigilance over years of experience.

2.1. Characteristics of pharmacovigilance in clinical trials

It is commonly known that not all hazards can be found before a drug is marketed. Pharmacovigilance is the science and activities relating to the detection, assessment, understanding and prevention of adverse effects or any other possible drug-related problems [12]. It is now also more involved in pre-approval drug assessment as well-designated clinical trials in phase IV, referred to "the clinical safety activities throughout the lifecycle of a medicinal product" [13]. Drugs at approval have limited clinical information from clinical trials. For example, 16,000 subjects are needed to receive a drug to detect one adverse drug event out of 10,000 people with 80% probability, while clinical trials for most new drugs are conducted with 2000–3000 patients prior to approval. Therefore, rare adverse drug reactions are hardly detected, although relatively common adverse drug reactions (ADRs) are identified. Patients with complex conditions are excluded in order to eliminate factors that may affect efficacy of a tested drug. Most, but not all, ADRs occur in rather short time after administration. The short duration of observation, for example, 1 year or less in clinical trials is another limitation that will not observe late-onset ADRs. CIOMS VI [13] would help readers understand systematic approach for safety management during clinical development. Missing information at approval concerning clinical safety often refers to use in children, elderly, kidney disorders, drugs for oncology, HIV, vaccines, biologicals, and other advanced drugs as they will all mostly have a comparatively small number of subjects. All those limitations are to be addressed in pharmacovigilance plan for post-marketing. Clinical trials need to be monitored by the Data and Safety Monitoring Boards (DSMBs), also known as Data Monitoring Committees (DMC), who periodically review and evaluate the accumulated data from one or multiple clinical trials for safety of trial subjects. After DSMB evaluation, apparently obvious favorable or unfavorable results in the treatment group will lead to recommendations to discontinue a trial for the reason of negative benefit-risk in the treatment of the control group. However, the benefit-risk assessment continues throughout the drug development lifecycle.

2.2. Hazard data collection: planning and practical realization

Although there are regulatory systems for both pre- and post-marketing individual case safety reports (ICSRs), the concept of cases to be reported is somewhat different between pre and post. After marketing, it is rather appropriate to pay more attention to unknown serious adverse reactions than known or non-serious ADRs, although the latter can provide useful supporting information about risk factors and nature of known ADRs. Clinical trials explore unknown properties and use of a medicine, and so taking ethics into account, all adverse events (AEs) must be collected and in addition, serious and unexpected adverse events are subject to expedited reporting.

All serious adverse events must be assessed regardless of causality by the applicant at the time of application submission. Furthermore, what kind of AE data can be collected in the development phase depends on the clinical evaluation stage in the development process in which the investigational drug is as described in the protocol. The judgment as to whether a case is expected (known) or unexpected (unknown) is based on the labeling of the marketed drug, while in clinical trials, the reference safety information in the investigator's brochure is used. It is necessary for clinical trial sponsors to update the investigator's brochure at any time as needed, and the latest reference safety information receives close regulatory attention to ensure it is up to date for the judgment of known/unknown (or listed/unlisted) cases.

In addition, since many of post-marketing ICSRs are spontaneous reports, there is a vast range in the quality of the information from rich cases to poor cases (e.g., age/gender, drug, and adverse event are minimum requirements for regulatory reporting), mostly without laboratory results and the exact size of the exposed population is unknown. Since laboratory test values of participants in a clinical trial are regularly collected, assessment of individual case safe report, described later in this chapter, should effectively utilize theses results for each subject as well as the corresponding case narratives. Clinical trials have detailed information on cases such as the AE development date and dose (details of which are often missing in post-marketing ICSRs) and the size of population is known, so it is possible to calculate the frequency of occurrence and the incidence of AE. Of course, efficacy is statistically evaluated in a prospective statistical analysis plan. Various designs of clinical investigation are available, not only clinical trials for the development of new drugs but also that for the extension of indication of existing drugs, development of new routes of administration, and changes in dosage regimen.

As regard to data collection of safety information in clinical trials, the Good Clinical Practice guideline [6] does not address details of standards for the types of data to be collected for safety monitoring although traditionally reliance has been placed mainly on AE case reporting to the regulatory agencies. While another guideline, ICH E2A [14], specify only the key data elements for inclusion in expedited reports of serious unexpected adverse drug reactions, it is prudent to collect more comprehensive safety data during development because poorly established safety profiles need to be clarified in greater detail with the collection of non-serious adverse events and essential laboratory data. Therefore, the study protocols should be well designed defining the data to be collected, which differs according to characteristics of a drug.

When collecting data, sponsors may prepare different procedures for targeted or untargeted AE detection. However, the methods are commonly used in the same manner such as questionnaires, patient diary cards, and medical records supplemented with serious adverse event (SAE) reporting forms. Safety outcomes can be presented using descriptive text or visual analogue scales for severity rating, based on subjective opinion, of adverse events during investigation, pre-, during-, and post-trial, since a participant was enrolled. Patients' opinions may not be scientifically presented, but an understanding of benefit and risk and impact of an AE on quality of life, thereby revitalizing patient-focused drug development, can be elaborated. Narratives are important information for in-depth investigation of suspected unexpected serious adverse drug reactions (SUSARs) and to understand the reasons why a participant has dropped out from a trial. A protocol needs to specify testing intervals and thresholds for evaluating data later. Discordance of coding interpreted from collected data will cause both false positives and false negatives. Issues of coding, if left unresolved, will worsen with multicenter research which will provide aggregate data for quantitative analysis.

How data are presented influences the impression that an assessor would have. An appropriate approach should be selected among many options such as tables with strata according to, for example, dosage, duration of treatment with scatter plots for clinical chemical data, Kaplan-Meier plots for cumulative hazard clinical chemical data and outcome evaluation, and so on.

2.3. Safety profile and risk assessment

It is important to gain an understanding of the safety profile of a drug as early and as much as possible during development as possible as risks can be more easily controlled. Once the efficacy is proven at the end of clinical development, the benefit-risk profile of the drug is reviewed whether it is acceptable for approval. Both medical judgment (qualitative) and statistics including descriptive and inferential approach (quantitative) influence the evaluation of clinical safety during drug development. The same principles apply to post-marketing evaluation. It is more likely, however, that safety signal detection and assessment during clinical development depend as much on clinical judgment with case reports, especially for serious rare AEs. Such an approach is reasonable and necessary for small-size trials, since data accumulation is limited due to the small number of subjects. With accumulated data, statistical methods are possibly available for the evaluation of safety signals in clinical trials, especially for more commonly occurring adverse events, and it is certainly a practical option to use a database for the phase IV studies especially after conditional approval has been granted. Any approaches need to consider patient population characteristics including natural history of disease and current therapeutic standards for comparison, when evaluating safety. Safety evaluation is the basis of risk assessment as a whole, and it is required to report an unusual or worrying ICSR, especially for AE of special interest, routinely anytime and when a certain evaluation milestone is reached such as with DSUR submissions.

Risk assessment as a part of pharmacovigilance in drug development requires analyzing and interpreting the safety profile. After risk assessment, investigator's brochure may be updated and risk management measures may be taken to minimize the risks, if necessary and medically significant. From perspectives of public health, risk assessment and decision-making should be done at the right time rather to wait for punctual dataset for review.

Although the clinical efficacy is steadily and iteratively demonstrated through phase I, II, and III, and then confirmed at the end of development, serious harm can occur at any stage of drug development. Thus pharmacovigilance in drug development may be more of a risk-based approach relating to any other drug-related issues that could affect patient safety and safe use of drug, including concerns about quality and efficacy as well as safety. In this sense, pharmacovigilance is consistent with a "risk-based approach" which to some extent can be found in regulatory guidances recently [15–17].

3. What can be done for "evaluating benefit-risk balance"?

Many methods have been proposed and each of them gives us thoughts to some extent. So, do we need to apply all to our daily work? Those evaluation methods have been reviewed in terms of usefulness in benefit-risk assessment and reported by the European Medicines Agency, suggesting three quantitative methods for regulatory assessment use, Bayesian statistics, Decision trees and influence/relevance diagrams and Multi-criteria analyses, as well as qualitative approach [18]. They also pointed out some limitations, for example, Bayesian statistical model do not generally deal with multiple criteria, and some other approaches such as conjoint analysis may contribute to some specific cases. An assessment process, which includes many dimensions of public health to consider, will be enforced by the integration of methods/approaches. Authors make the point that quantitative methods/approaches are effectively adopted in practice only when a qualitative approach works.

3.1. Basic processes of adverse event evaluation

The identification of a potential safety issue for a drug requires processes to distinguish adverse reactions from unrelated adverse events. These cases can be found in reports submitted to regulatory authorities or published articles/posts through journals, media and even through social media and Internet. As a basic reference for risk assessment, the evaluation result of each individual case of suspected ADRs, as well as adverse events, is important because even one ADR case can be sufficient by evidence itself of a risk serious enough to stop a clinical trial. Therefore, the first step of the process is the assessment of individual case observations, and the difficulties of causality assessment are addressed further in the next Section 3.2. Case evaluation needs to consider clinical significance, seriousness, severity (continuous variables), and expectedness based on the latest investigator's brochure, causality, place and time of occurrence, dosage, and predisposing factors of trial subject. AEs based on laboratory data need to be interpreted as to whether they are of value as surrogate markers, whether testing intervals are adequate and whether such surrogate markers can be correlated with or help predict harmful endpoints.

Detection of specific ADRs as harmful properties of a medicine itself has an obvious purpose. These can be grouped or aggregate cases with features in common or a case series where the number of cases, individual causalities, inter-case consistency, and severity/seriousness can all be assessed. Plausibility of causal relationship between a drug and event can be discussed on the ground of causal assessment of each case or of a group of cases as an aggregate.

The next stage for attributing causality is to review the statistical quantification of safety data from individual studies. Biostatisticians can prepare and present data with tables and graphics as well as quantities of continuous/discrete variables. Points to consider include epidemiological morbidity and subjects' background data (bias and confounders), investigational comparators, randomization or not, primary/secondary/surrogate endpoint, dropouts and missing data, and data dependency on dose and time (hazard function). All aspects of statistical testing may play a critical role when applying a statistical analysis plan: types of test, probability threshold (p-level), adjustment for multiple testing and confounders, power of test, and confident intervals.

Toward the end of development, all data pooled through clinical trials are reviewed. This may require meta-analysis of individual data of clinical trials as well as meta-analysis of published studies as well. It has been reported that no significant difference exists between meta-analysis of published data and of individual data, and using published data is still considered the norm [19]. From different studies, there needs to be a pooling of numerators (e.g., number of affected patients) and denominators (e.g., number of patients or patient years) for ADR frequency estimation; frequency expression as "number needed to treat to harm," pooling of within-study and between-treatment group differences.

After AE assessment, if necessary, a sponsor should update the investigator's brochure and continue developing the labeling and future surveillance plan. Accordingly, Core Safety Information of an investigator's brochure should be based on the Company Core Safety Information, which in turn will be transferred to the Summary of Product Characteristics. To extend development, phase IV studies are possible, for example, with registers for long-term follow-up, observational studies for safety in clinical setting or using the large clinical database.

3.2. Qualitative data: case narrative

Many algorithms and classification systems on causality have been proposed; however, none has been agreed and accepted by everyone. In recent years, it has been questioned whether it is worthwhile to spend much effort conducting causality assessment on individual suspected ADR reports. The reason why is that ICSRs are considered relatively weaker as an evidence for causality than compared to the frequency of events in the actively treated group with that of the comparative control group. If randomized controlled trials found significant differences with appropriate statistical power, it is likely that pharmacotherapy was the cause of event, that is, the medicinal product directly caused the event under certain conditions of use. It is important to ensure robustness and objectivity of the trial is preserved by blinding (as qualitative assessment of unblinded data is considered subjective). But can even the best conduct clinical trials replace spontaneous reporting? Clinical trials from the early development phase to phase IV cannot replace spontaneous ADR reporting systems for detecting very rare ADRs, and it is not realistic to conduct a large-scale epidemiological survey/study for each new drug. Large databases may consider a signal such a rare ADR as noise and so it may be missed. Therefore, even though information technology has evolved, it remains important to evaluate causal relationship qualitatively on ICSRs individually, using medical inference, taking into account the widely different circumstances in which they arise ranging from clinical trials, registries, to spontaneous reports.

As a tool to assist qualitative evaluation, A to F ADR classes have been proposed and extended since the 1970s. It addresses the characteristics of how to categorize ADRs pharmacologically: Type A—augmented; Type B—bizarre; Type C—chronic; Type D—delayed; Type E—end of use; and Type F—failure of therapy [20, 21].

In addition, the DoTS classification considering dose, time, and susceptibility was also proposed from the viewpoint of elements that are thought to affect how side effects become manifested rather than the pathology of side effects in isolation (**Table 1**). [21] The authors recognize absorption/distribution/metabolism/elimination to be included as susceptibility factors and, in addition, propose to consider these factors as contributing to medication error (contribution of human factors and other causal and predisposing factors).

WHO-Uppsala Monitoring Center advises that evaluation of causality can be categorized into six stages, such as certain, probable, possible, unlikely, conditional/unclassified, and unassessable/unclassifiable [22], and for that the following major four aspects are to be considered [23]. (1) temporal relationships: What is the temporal relationship between treatment initiation and the beginning of the event? How has the event changed after discontinuing treatment? (negative dechallenge) Did it recur after re-administration? (positive rechallenge) (2) Alternative causes: Have there been exposure factors other than complications, concomitant medications, or medicines that can explain the event occurrence? (3) Nature of the event: Some clinical events are often caused immediately by drugs (e.g., swelling in injection site). (4) Plausibility: Is the reaction already recognized by this medicine? (Is it a known side effect with this class?) Can the explanation for mechanism of event be derived from its known pharmacological action?

As a more specific evaluation criterion, nine criteria by Hill [24] and a number of scoring algorithms such as that devised by Naranjo et al. [25] can be used and applied to as part of causality assessment. Effective use of all these causality techniques requires practical knowledge about how to blend clinical, medical, and pharmacological sciences, which it means it is necessary to have suitably qualified persons with such knowledge actively leading and involved in the assessment team. Behavioral competencies for effective performance in pharmacovigilance have been discussed elsewhere [26].

As will be described later, it is not uncommon for elucidation of the mechanism of the development of ADR after many years following new drug approval often linked to advances in in scientific technology and research. Benefit-risk assessment that involves scientific review should be considered as standard operational procedures with structured framework to achieve feasible decision-making. However, as there are no perfect causality criteria, we should always bear in mind and not ignore clinical significant events regardless of causality unless there is overwhelming evidence of other causal factors which are obvious.

Dose	Time	Susceptibility
Toxic	Time independent	Age
Collateral	Time dependent (rapid, first dose, and early/intermediate/ late/delayed)	Sex
Hypersusceptibility		Physiological variation
		Exogenous factors
		Disease

Table 1. DoTS classification of adverse drug reaction.

http://dx.doi.org/10.5772/intechopen.76331

3.3. Quantitative data: statistical approach

Statistics are widely used in the drug development as "biostatistics" to validate the efficiency of investigational products entity. What about the application of statistics to assess safety?

In the mid-1980s, the term "pharmacoepidemiology" was used for the first time, which often refers to the academic field of study, drug use and safety on a group level. As you can imagine from the phrase "epidemiology," the "group of subjects" or "population" studied by pharmacoepidemiology is a larger patient group than that of the clinical trial numbering up to tens of thousands or even an entire national population. This academic field has greatly expanded in the 1990s which is underpinned by the increased use of computerized databases including prescription records and clinical outcomes to investigate safety issues quickly and efficiently, as well as sophisticated computer technology, which enables high-enough performance to handle enormous amounts of data.

More recently, the design of pharmacoepidemiologic studies has turned to using big data. No matter the size of study subjects, the most challenging aspect of pharmacoepidemiology is its research design as with clinical trials. The place of "chance" that may lead statistically significant difference, "Bias" by systematic error, and "Confounding" as a third factor associated with both drugs and events, all may contribute to a direct association between drugs and events, which should be considered when designing the research plan and considering their results. Studies on drug safety are often performed further in the post-marketing phase observationally. Because, a double-blind trial to verify whether a serious adverse event will occur to a patient can be ethically dubious as patients cannot be denied an approved effective medicine, and in order to mitigate weakness and strengthen observational studies, pharmacoepidemiological researches inevitably consider new designs. In this academic domain, study designs and statistical techniques have been evolved, such as self-controlled case series, new user design, etc., handling bias and confounding that are classic and common in cohort and case-control studies. Frequently used study designs in pharmacoepidemiology are described further in the regulatory guidelines and the academic proposals [27–29].

New designs seem to be developed and used mainly for retrospective observational database studies. For the question of interest, there is still needs to conduct a traditional epidemiological study design for post-approval, phase IV study. As with the example of Brigham and Women's Hospital epidemiological studies, it may be necessary to plan for a cohort study to assemble from the beginning of development. Recently, many large-scale databases are becoming available and it is prudent to first make use of them. When choosing a database, you should make sure that prescription records, event data, and health-related information, such as gender and age, are available. If you can reconcile patient ID, separate databases may be combined. However, this requires epidemiological knowledge and experience.

3.4. Much to do in the post-marketing phase to fully develop and define a medicine's properties and potential

Based on the principle of ICH E2E, risk management plans have become a part of a new drug approval document to be submitted to the regulatory authorities in many countries/regions.

Most of the processes for evaluating ADRs are similar in the pre- and post-authorization phases, although differences are found in data source for evaluation which impact on the quality and meaning of an adverse event case. One of the significant differences is that the spontaneous reporting system plays a critical role in post-authorization for both qualitative and quantitative analysis, especially for the identification of potential safety issues as soon as possible. This requires the process for quality management of spontaneous reporting so that spontaneous reporting to be improved [30].

One of major challenges of ICSR reporting is its quality variation over time and between different geographical regions, depending on reporting cultures and regulations. This means it is to be expected that the databases of aggregated ICSRs can vary between countries/regions and indicate different drug-event combinations as safety signals. To illustrate these differences, a comparison study was performed on ICSRs databases between the United States and Japan, namely, FDA Adverse Events Reporting System (FAERS) and Japanese Adverse Drug Event Report (JADER) [31]. The ICSR elements and their definitions defined by ICH have been implemented by countries/regions. It is expected that a case should be recorded in the same manner in different countries, however, not in reality. In the study, although both databases limitedly open the data elements, there were discrepancies in the type of reported AEs, reported drugs, reporter type, seriousness, and average number of reported events per case, between the JADER and FAERS. For example, the average number of AEs per case was 1.6 (SD = 1.3, max = 37) in the JADER and 3.3 (SD = 3.5, max = 62) for the Japanese cases in the FAERS; "drug exposure during pregnancy," "no adverse events," and non-serious cases are present in FAERS, but as these are not mandatory for electronic submission in Japan, few reports from non-professionals were found in the JADER.

These differences are mostly due to regulations and customs. In addition to these, social factors and healthcare systems also have a considerable impact. Interstitial lung disease (ILD) is an example of how an AE can be differently reported in Japan based on social-induced reporting bias. Japan has experienced serious social concerns with ILD related to several drugs and simultaneously, diagnosis with x-ray imaging is available in Japanese clinics and hospitals so it would appear that ILD could be more efficiently detected than other countries. Coding rules also may affect ICSRs data, because medical terminologies of ICSRs are submitted using codes inputted by a reporting company, where the company culture may have been embedded in the process so that bias may arise. All these unresolved biases threaten internal and external validity of the ICSR databases.

Nevertheless, the ICSR database is still very useful for review in the post-approval phase. It gives an opportunity to detect any safety signal (a combination of a medicine and an event considered to require more detailed examination) that would require a closer scrutiny. Collecting individual cases in the post-approval phase is said to be particularly suited for capturing suspected cases of serious and rare adverse drug reactions; however, if healthcare professionals, especially physicians, do not report the event, the potential safety risk cannot be noticed. In order to complement this, those who evaluate actively post-marketing data are extending their activities to include looking for signals from a large amount of information, which is out of scope of this chapter.

Data management and statistical methods draw attention to the need to press forward by improving the efficiency of data analysis. However, it is hard for database analyses to identify issues such as dependency problems of medicines such as benzodiazepines and many delayed side effects unless they are flagged as a safety problem by patients' complaints in the first place through spontaneous reporting.

4. Remaining issues and the future for pharmacovigilance

4.1. Characteristics of phase IV studies

Phase IV studies, either interventional or observational studies, have to be appropriately designed, according to the purpose/hypothesis about drug efficacy, effectiveness, or safety. To say that "the medicine is safe" in regulatory science means that the probability of hazard is low and acceptable, as compared to the disease to be treated and the benefit expected by the drug. In that sense, the safety concerns of the marketed drug are always linked to the benefit of the drug which has been accepted in the approval process. Unlike "efficacy" review, observational studies prevail in drug safety due to ethical reasons. Clinical trials are designed to reduce a statistical erroneous conclusion that efficacy exists when it really does not (Type I error). It defines "efficacy" to be tested, and statistical analysis is planned on the basis of a single hypothesis of the efficacy, thus the testing of multiple hypothesis within a single study is discouraged. However, there are a lot of potential types of ADRs that would be inappropriate to examine in a randomized trial. This is another reason for using surveillance to catch any signs of hazard and using prospective/retrospective longitudinal observational studies and pharmacoepidemiological database studies to assess the occurrence of ADRs. In addition, population-based design is of significance to compensate limited generalizability in clinical trials. "Effectiveness" in real-world clinical settings of a drug is scrutinized normally by non-interventional study or trial where the drugs are prescribed as per usual based on the terms of a drug marketing license. Definition of "effectiveness" may be prone to chance of subjective variation of the prescribing physician, which would make designing a study difficult.

Some registration systems provide an overview of clinical trials and studies: purpose, study type, intervention, recruitment criteria, etc. One such system in regulatory use is ClinicalTrials.gov, where information on phase II to IV studies of drugs, biological products, and medical devices regulated by the FDA is submitted [32–34]. Approximately 20,000 phase IV studies, over a half of which were interventional, have been registered in ClinicalTrials.gov; among over 250,000 studies in 203 countries, noticeably, registered phase IV studies include studies without drugs and observational studies [35, 36]. Those interventional studies examine various aspects of efficacy, pharmacodynamics, pharmacokinetics and other pharmacological aspects. Safety is often focused along with efficacy as described above, and 4392 of 4722 safety studies were aimed at efficacy as well as safety from 2004 to 2014. Of those which were interventional studies, 226 (68.5%) of them recruited less than 300 patients. Again, from a public health view point of generalizability, safety profile cannot be efficiently informed through clinical studies alone.

4.2. Utilizing and making sense of new data sources

Real world data (RWD) refers to all the data relating to patient health status and/or the delivery of health care routinely collected from a variety of sources [37]. They are collected under day-to-day circumstances and not through international trials with a control or comparative group. This means data are outside the controlled constraints of conventional randomized clinical trials. Especially occurring in the post-approval setting, the data can be used to evaluate what happens when a medicine is used in normal clinical practice. Such data can arise from a number of sources, not only in the clinical settings, but also social settings. Therefore, RWD can be found in electronic health records (EHRs), claims and billing activities, product and disease registries, patient-related activities in out-patient or in-home use settings, health-monitoring devices and even blogs if possible [38]. In addition, RWD can include data on outcomes (both clinical and patient-reported), resource use (medical institutions, patient, and societal), treatment pathways, service models, patient preference, experience, and compliance. Secondary research data derived from routinely collected data is also applicable. Real-world evidence in drug development is, in turn, the clinical evidence regarding the usage and potential benefits or risks of a medical product derived from the analysis of all of this RWD.

RWD and RWE may not be the best thing for collecting efficacy data, and interventional trials are essential and inevitable to prove efficacy of medicinal entity. The methodology to utilize RWD would elaborate the better use of RWD for the monitoring of safety information in the post-approval phase to add further information on benefit-risk balance [39]. As of today, the majority of studies with RWD are safety-focused, and real-world pharmacovigilance is one of the main drivers currently for collection of RWD for many companies, based on post-authorization requirements for safety evaluation in real-world patients. It is reported that registries, in the form of a cohort study, have not sufficiently enrolled participants [40], and it should bear in mind that any type of data source has difficulties and limitations in collection and quality of its data.

4.3. Necessity of pharmacovigilance for the development of pharmaceuticals

Access to new therapies in oncology has depended on the results of post-approval RWD. There are some drugs approved based on progression-free survival using Kaplan-Meier survival analysis with no difference in overall survival time. Can the data of progression-free survival really support a clinically meaningful effect of anticancer drugs? Would not data about the overall survival period be better? It may be agreed with regulators that data on the overall survival time derived from post-approval observational research be evaluated with the results fed back to healthcare professionals through updates to the package insert, etc. Such an approach may well lead to increase in utilization of conditional approvals.

Beginning with imatinib, the development of molecular-targeted drugs and utilization in clinical practice became popular especially in the twenty-first century. However, it has been noted in recent years that many genetic mutations are present in the signal transduction system and from this scientist can more easily predict outcomes concerning effectiveness and safety. Even though we cannot fully clarify molecular targeted drugs at the time of approval, research for confirming gene mutation should continue to be recommended after marketing by using companion diagnostic agents often as personalized medicine. As the tragedy of thalidomide was one milestone, the lessons learned after gefitinib's marketing in Japan can be considered a further milestone for molecular targeted drugs. Gefitinib was the second molecular-targeted drug that was launched in Japan ahead of the world in July 2002 based on the approved indication of lung cancer. Some years later, it was confirmed that the effectiveness is valid for small cell lung cancer patients with EGFR gene mutation (L858R or Exon 19 deficiency), and that the mutation of the ATP binding site is more common in Oriental women such as Japan and China [41]. In terms of safety, many adverse reaction cases of Interstitial Lung Disease were reported at the time of clinical trials, but the mechanism of action that caused such an adverse reaction had not yet been elucidated.

However, there remains a huge question about the feasibility for a company being obliged to obtain even more data during development by investing in post-marketing safety studies and effectiveness studies. In recent years, regulatory authorities have streamlined reviews for approval, such as FDA's Accelerated Approval Program, and there are increasing numbers of applications requiring post-approval safety measures at the time of approval. It is considered as one possible solution to replace conducting many phase IV studies and in vitro studies with utilizing RWD, as described above. However, it should be noted that profiles of each database vary so much that they produce different results even if you study with the same objective, for example, pioglitazone [42]. Therefore, it is necessary to sufficiently clarify the risk minimization actions in a RMP, and to keep these in mind when choosing a database for quantitative assessment.

5. Conclusions

Pharmacovigilance can be defined as a multidisciplinary science consisting of systematic activities and processes relating to the detection, assessment, understanding, and prevention of adverse effects or any other problems related to medical healthcare products and their handling throughout their lifecycle, thus mitigating risk and maximizing benefits for patients. These activities include those required to monitor and assess a quality system embedded in a just and fair culture that facilitates reporting, communication, and organizational learning to demonstrate that the system is performing according to guiding safety principles agreed by all stakeholders. What has been learned from the history of various medicines is that the balance between benefit and risk can change from time to time based on the obtained experience and information, and that taking multiple approaches to a certain safety research objective can often result in different answers. Therefore, pharmacovigilance is a challenging and evolving multidisciplinary science that has to be applied logically throughout drug lifecycle. This chapter presented what are available in practice to assess and profile safety with a central aspect of adverse drug event/reaction throughout the development phase to the post-marketing phase.

Conflict of interest

No potential conflict of interest was reported by the authors.

Author details

Kaori Nomura[1*] and Brian David Edwards[2]

*Address all correspondence to: kaori.nomura@jikei.ac.jp

1 Jikei University School of Medicine, Tokyo, Japan

2 NDA Regulatory Science Ltd, London, UK

References

[1] Pirmohamed M, Park K. Adverse drug reactions: Back to the future. British Journal of Clinical Pharmacology. 2003;**55**:486-492

[2] Waller P. An Introduction to Pharmacovigilance. Chichester: John Wiley & Sons Ltd.; 2010. 3 p. DOI: 10.1002/9781444316766

[3] Kerbrat A, Ferre JC, Fillatre P, et al. Acute neurologic disorder from an inhibitor of fatty acid amide hydrolase. The New England Journal of Medicine. 2016;**375**:1717-1725. DOI: 10.1056/NEJMoa1604221

[4] International Conference on Harmonisation of the Technical Requirements for Registration of Pharmaceuticals for Human Use. ICH Harmonised Tripartite Guideline E6 Guideline for Good Clinical Practice [Internet]. 1996. Available from: https://www.ich.org/fileadmin/Public_Web_Site/ICH_Products/Guidelines/Efficacy/E6/E6_R1_Guideline.pdf [Accessed: Feb 1, 2018]

[5] Council for International Organizations of Medical Sciences. Report of CIOMS Working Group VII: The Development Safety Update Report (DSUR): Harmonizing the Format and Content for Periodic Safety Reporting During Clinical Trials. Geneva: Council for International Organizations of Medical Sciences; 2006

[6] International Conference on Harmonisation of Technical Requirements for Registration of Pharmaceuticals for Human Use. ICH Harmonised Tripartite Guideline E2F Development Safety Update Report [Internet]. 2005. Available from: http://www.ich.org/fileadmin/Public_Web_Site/ICH_Products/Guidelines/Efficacy/E2F/Step4/E2F_Step_4.pdf [Accessed: Feb 1, 2018]

[7] International Organization for Standardization. ISO31000:2009 Risk Management – Principles and Guidelines. [Internet] 2009. Available from: https://www.iso.org/obp/ui/#iso:std:iso:31000:ed-1:v1:en [Accessed: 15 April 2018]

[8] International Organization for Standardization. ISO14971:2007 Medical Devices – Application of Risk Management to Medical Devices. [Internet] 2007. Available from: https://www.iso.org/obp/ui/#iso:std:iso:14971:ed-2:v2:en:sec:H [Accessed: 15 April 2018]

[9] International Conference on Harmonisation of Technical Requirements for Registration of Pharmaceuticals for Human Use. Q9 Quality Risk Management [Internet]. 2005. Available from: http://www.ich.org/fileadmin/Public_Web_Site/ICH_Products/Guidelines/Quality/Q9/Step4/Q9_Guideline.pdf [Accessed: Feb 1, 2018]

[10] Directive 2001/83/EC of the European Parliament and of the Council of 6 November 2001 on the Community Code Relating to Medicinal Products for Human Use. (as amended) [Internet]. Available from https://ec.europa.eu/health/sites/health/files/files/eudralex/vol-1/dir_2001_83_consol_2012/dir_2001_83_cons_2012_en.pdf [Accessed: Feb 1, 2018]

[11] Lindquist M. The need for definitions in pharmacovigilance. Drug Safety. 2007;**30**(10): 825-830. DOI: 0114-5916/07/0010-0825/$44.95/0

[12] World Health Organization. The Importance of Pharmacovigilance – Safety Monitoring of Medicinal Products. Geneva: World Health Organization; 2002

[13] Council for International Organizations of Medical Sciences. Report of CIOMS Working Group VI: Management of Safety Information from Clinical Trials. Geneva: Council for International Organizations of Medical Sciences. 2005

[14] International Conference on Harmonisation of Technical Requirements for Registration of Pharmaceuticals for Human Use. E2A Clinical Safety Data Management: Definitions and Standards for Expedited Reporting [Internet]. 1994. Available from: https://www.ich.org/fileadmin/Public_Web_Site/ICH_Products/Guidelines/Efficacy/E2A/Step4/E2A_Guideline.pdf [Accessed: Feb 1, 2018]

[15] European Medicines Agency. Guideline on the Risk-based Approach According to Annex I, Part IV of Directive 2001/83/EC Applied to Advanced Therapy Medicinal Products [Internet]. Feb 11, 2013. Available from: http://www.ema.europa.eu/docs/en_GB/document_library/Scientific_guideline/2013/03/WC500139748.pdf [Accessed: Feb 1, 2018]

[16] European Medicines Agency. Reflection Paper on Risk-based Quality Management in Clinical Trials [Internet]. Nov 18, 2013. Available from: http://www.ema.europa.eu/docs/en_GB/document_library/Scientific_guideline/2013/11/WC500155491.pdf [Accessed: Feb 1, 2018]

[17] Food and Drug Administration. Guidance for Industry Oversight of Clinical Investigations – A Risk-based Approach to Monitoring [Internet]. August 2013. Available from: https://www.fda.gov/downloads/Drugs/Guidances/UCM269919.pdf [Accessed: Feb 1, 2018]

[18] European Medicines Agency. 2010. European Medicines Agency. Benefit-risk Methodology Project Work Package 2 Report: Applicability of Current Tools and Processes for Regulatory Benefit-risk Assessment [Internet]. Aug 31, 2013. Available from: http://www.ema.europa.eu/docs/en_GB/document_library/Report/2010/10/WC500097750.pdf [Accessed: Feb 1, 2018]

[19] Angelillo IF, Villari P. Meta-analysis of published studies or meta-analysis of individual data? Caesarean section in HIV-positive women as a study case. Public Health. 2003 Sep;**117**(5):323-328. DOI: 10.1016/S0033-3506(03)00105-7

[20] Rawlins MD. Clinical pharmacology: Adverse reactions to drugs. British Medical Journal. 1981;**282**:974-976 [Internet]. Available from: https://www.ncbi.nlm.nih.gov/pmc/articles/PMC1504743/pdf/bmjcred00650-0048.pdf [Accessed: Feb 1, 2018]

[21] Aronson JK, Ferner RE. Joining the DoTS: New approach to classifying adverse drug reactions. British Medical Journal. 2003;**327**:1222-1227. DOI: 10.1136/bmj.327.7425.1222

[22] Uppsala Monitoring Center. The Use of the WHO-UMC System for Standardised Case Causality Assessment [Internet]. Available from: http://www.who.int/medicines/areas/quality_safety/safety_efficacy/WHOcausality_assessment.pdf [Accessed: Feb 1, 2018]

[23] Waller P. An Introduction to Pharmacovigilance. Chichester: John Wiley & Sons Ltd.; 2010. 25-27 p. DOI: 10.1002/9781444316766

[24] Hill AB. The environment and disease: Association or causation? Proceedings of the Royal Society of Medicine. 1965;**58**(5):295-300

[25] Naranjo CA, Busto U, Sellars EA, et al. A method for estimating the probability of adverse drug reactions. Clinical Pharmacology and Therapeutics. 1981;**30**:239-245. DOI: 10.1038/clpt.1981.154

[26] Edwards B, Tilson HH, West SL. Defining the competencies of those conducting pharmacovigilance. Pharmacoepidemiology and Drug Safety. 2006;**15**(3):193-198. DOI: 10.1002/pds.1153

[27] FDA. Structured Approach to Benefit-Risk Assessment in Drug Regulatory Decision-Making [Internet]. 2013. Available from: https://www.fda.gov/downloads/forindustry/userfees/prescriptiondruguserfee/ucm329758.pdf [Accessed: Feb 14, 2018]

[28] European Medicines Agency. The European Network of Centres for Pharmacoepidemiology and Pharmacovigilance (ENCePP) Guide on Methodological Standards in Pharmacoepidemiology (Revision 6) [Internet]. 2010. Available from: http://www.encepp.eu/standards_and_guidances/documents/ENCePPGuideofMethStandardsinPE_Rev6.pdf [Accessed: Feb 14, 2018]

[29] International Society for Pharmacoepidemiology. Guidelines for Good Pharmacoepidemiology Practices (GPP) [Internet]. 2015. Available from: https://www.pharmacoepi.org/resources/policies/guidelines-08027/. [Accessed: Feb 14, 2018]

[30] Prabhakar U, Edwards B. Postmarketing safety surveillance issues with data collection for postmarketing pharmacovigilance. Pharmaceutical Medicine. 2010;**24**(6):343-348. DOI: 10.1007/BF03256835

[31] Nomura K, Takahashi K, Hinomura Y, et al. Effect of database profile variation on drug safety assessment: An analysis of spontaneous adverse event reports of Japanese cases. Drug Design, Development and Therapeutics. 2015;**9**:3031-3041. DOI: 10.2147/DDDT.S81998

[32] Gillen JE, Tse T, Ide NC, McCray AT. Design, implementation and management of a web-based data entry system for ClinicalTrials.gov. Studies in Health Technology and Informatics. 2004;**107**(Pt 2):1466-1470. DOI: 10.3233/978-1-60750-949-3-1466

[33] Zarin DA, Keselman A. Registering a clinical trial in ClinicalTrials.gov. Chest. 2007;**131**(3):909-912. DOI: https://doi.org/10.1378/chest.06-2450

[34] Tse T, Williams RJ, Zarin DA. Update on registration of clinical trials in ClinicalTrials.gov. Chest. 2009;**135**:304-305. DOI: 10.1378/chest.09-1219

[35] U.S. National Library of Medicine. [Internet]. Available from: https://clinicaltrials.gov [Accessed: Feb 14, 2018]

[36] Zhang X, Zhang Y, Ye X, et al Overview of phase IV clinical trials for postmarket drug safety surveillance: A status report from the ClinicalTrials.gov registry. BMJ Open. 2016;6:e010643. DOI: 10.1136/bmjopen-2015-010643

[37] Food and Drug Administration. Real World Evidence. 2018. Available from: https://www.fda.gov/scienceresearch/specialtopics/realworldevidence/default.htm

[38] Sherman, RE, Anderson, SA, Dal Pan, GJ et al. Real-world evidence – What is it and what can it tell us?. The New England Journal of Medicine; 2016:**375**(23):2293-2297p. DOI: 10.1056/NEJMsb1609216

[39] Goldman M. The Valuable World of Real World Evidence [Internet]. 2014. Available from: http://www.pharmafile.com/news/196159/valuable-world-real-world-evidence. [Accessed: Feb 14, 2018]

[40] Bouvy JC, Blake K, Slattery J, et al. Registries in European post-marketing surveillance: A retrospective analysis of centrally approved products, 2005-2013. Pharmacoepidemiology and Drug Safety. 2017;**26**(12):1442-1450. DOI: 10.1002/pds.4196

[41] Morita S, Okamoto I, Kobayashi K, et al. Combined survival analysis of prospective clinical trials of gefitinib for non-small cell lung cancer with EGFR mutations. Clinical Cancer Research. 2009;**15**(13):4493-4498. DOI: 10.1158/1078-0432.CCR-09-0391

[42] Filipova E, Uzunova K, Kalinov K, Vekov T. Pioglitazone and the risk of bladder cancer: A meta-analysis. Diabetes Therapy. 2017;**8**(4):705-726. DOI: 10.1007/s13300-017-0273-4

Chapter 3

Integrated Approach to Nature as Source of New Drug Lead

Seema Kohli

Additional information is available at the end of the chapter

http://dx.doi.org/10.5772/intechopen.74961

Abstract

Classically, the development and launching of a new drug is a highly time consuming, tedious and expensive process involving following fundamental steps: (1) Identification of cause of Disease and Search for target site. (2) Search and Optimisation of active compound, that is, the Drug Lead. (3) Testing of Drug in Animals (pre-clinical phase). (4) Clinical Trials. (5) Approval of New Drug by Competent authority and availability of the drug. Drug discovery and development process involves around 10–15 years of investigation period and incredibly high cost and investment. This process also involves participation of experts from various disciplines and fields. Therefore, the new approaches are obligatory to be developed not only to expedite the process but also to ensure the launch of safer and effective drug. Over this background, the importance of experimental wisdom and holistic approach is intensifying to offer good base as an attractive discovery engine. Natural product drug discovery, ethno-pharmacology, traditional and attractive medicines are re-emerging as new strategic options. In the past decade, the number of new chemical entity (NCG) in drug development channel is declining markedly might have led to the rekindling of interest in emergence of natural product as new drug leads. The novel natural products can be optimised on the basis of their biological activities using highly sophisticated combinatorial biosynthetic techniques, microbial genomes and screening process.

Keywords: natural products, drug leads, microorganism and marine source

1. Introduction

Drug discovery and development is mainly concerned with new chemical entity with biological activity. It works on enhancing the properties of drugs used in the treatment of different medical conditions. Classically, the development and launching of a new drug is a highly time-consuming, tedious and expensive process involving under mentioned fundamental steps:

- Identification of cause of Disease and Search for target site
- Search and Optimisation of active compound, that is, the Drug Lead
- Testing of Drug in Animals (pre-clinical phase)
- Clinical Trials
- Approval of New Drug by Competent authority and availability in market.

Drug discovery leading to strong and doable lead candidate always remained exigent assignment for scientists. In fact experts accomplish the task by transforming the screening hit compound to a suitable drug candidate. The journey of new drug to the market is considerably long and takes about 10–15 years of investigation period. Therefore, the new approaches are obligatory to be developed not only to expedite the process but also to ensure the launch of safer and effective drug [1].

Over this background, the importance of experimental wisdom and holistic approach is intensifying to offer good base as an attractive discovery engine. Natural product drug discovery, ethno-pharmacology, traditional and attractive medicines are re-emerging as new strategic options. In the past decade, the number of new chemical entity (NCE) in drug development channel is declining markedly might have led to the rekindling of interest in the emergence of natural product new drug leads. The novel-natural products can be optimised on the basis of their biological activities using highly sophisticated combinatorial biosynthetic techniques, microbial genomes and screening process (**Figure 1**).

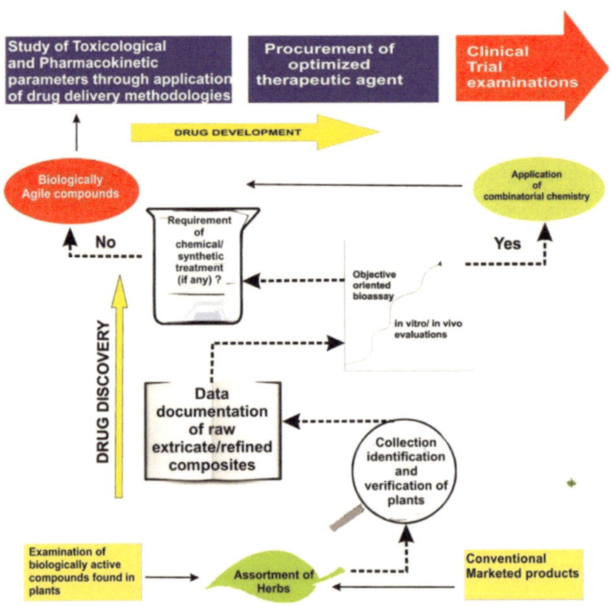

Figure 1. Complete process of drug discovery from plants.

Since ages the natural products have been the source of medicinal agents and will continue to play crucial role in the human health through the expanded investigation of world biodiversity. World Health Organization (WHO) reports that about 80% of the world's population depends on traditional medicine for their health care. Further, at least 119 important chemical substances have been derived from 90 plant species [2].

With the advent of theory of drug-receptor action, the scientists concluded that it is the isolated compound from the plant extract that is responsible for pharmacological action. This leads to new era in pharmacology and area of new drug research. The classical example is morphine (from opium) and digoxin (from *Digitalis purpurea*). A number of modern medicines have been obtained from natural resources such as plants, microorganisms, marine organisms and minerals. Nature continues to be a main source of molecular diversity, which through the pursuit of multidisciplinary, international collaborative research can result in the development of promising lead compounds [3].

2. Natural product as new drug lead

Lead identification/optimisation is the one of the most important steps in drug development following the biological target identification. The properties of a drug can be enhanced or potentiated by making certain modifications/alterations in its chemical structure. Drug efficacy, potency, selectivity and pharmacokinetic parameters can be improved by making necessary structural changes. The chemical structure is the key to lead compound identification. After the lead compound identification, the next step is the study of ADMET that is absorption, distribution, metabolism, excertion and toxicology of the probable drug lead. If these studies are positive and satisfactory, the compound is nontoxic and non-mutagenic, then the compound is turned to be potential lead compound. This may then be developed as new drug. (**Figure 2**). Lead compound is a chemical compound that shows desired pharmacological activity and may initiate the development of new chemical entity, relevant compound. These are actually the starting molecule for the new drug. Newer techniques can be adopted to accelerate the enhancement in the compounds pharmacological properties.

The promising sources of lead compound and novel drugs are:

- Natural products
- Chemical libraries
- Computational Medicinal Chemistry

Recently, there has been a keen interest in natural product research as the traditional method of drug discovery failed to yield desired lead compound particularly in areas such as immunosuppressant, anti-infective and metabolic diseases. Natural product research continues to explore a variety of lead chemical structures that can be used as a template for new drug by the pharmaceutical industry. This is also evident that new approaches to enhance the joint drug discovery and development process would be expected to take place basically from

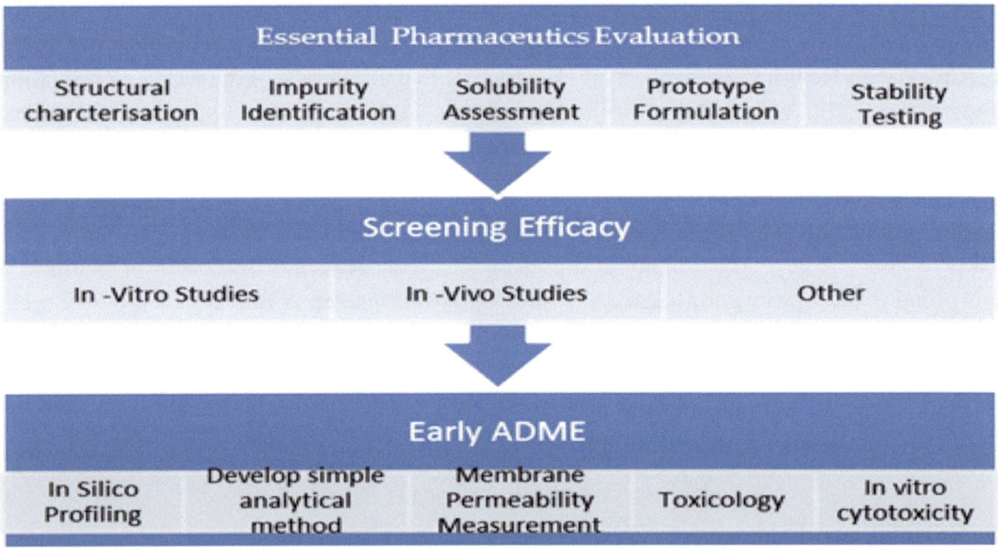

Figure 2. Process of lead selections and identification.

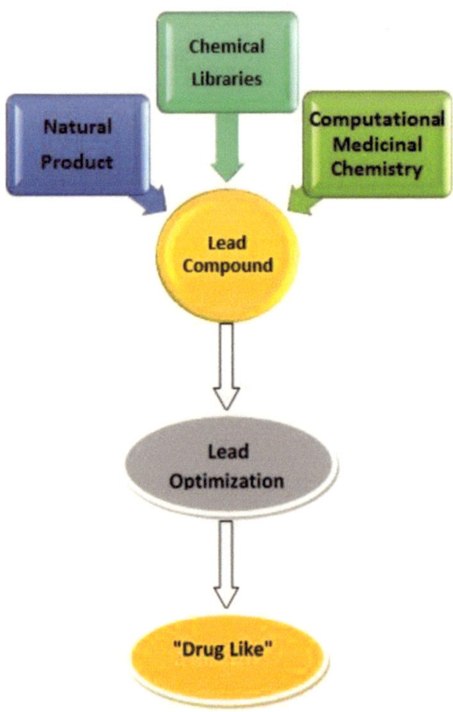

Figure 3. Drug leads and drug development.

innovation in drug target elucidation along with lead structure discovery. There are new technologies like automated separation techniques, high throughput screening and combinatorial chemistry are powerful and revolutionising drug discovery. (**Figure 3**).

http://dx.doi.org/10.5772/intechopen.74961

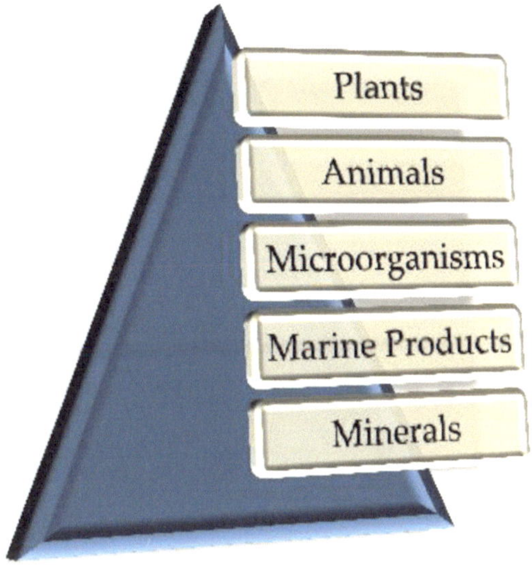

Figure 4. Natural products as drug leads.

Apart from comparing with other drug discovery methods, natural products are still providing their fair share of new clinical candidates and drugs. These said compounds were still a significant source of new drugs, especially in the anticancer, anti-infective, antihypertensive, immune-suppression and neurological disease therapeutic areas [4–7]. The natural products used as drug lead are shown in **Figure 4**.

2.1. Plants

Plants are affluent source of pharmaceuticals as well as drug leads. They are the natural laboratories where the simple chemical skeleton is transformed to complex chemical structures. The natural metabolites are far better than the synthesised metabolites in biological efficacy. A survey of plant-derived drugs in countries that host the WHO—Traditional medicinal Centres indicated that out of 122 compound identified 80% were derived from 94 plant species. Some of the drugs obtained in this approach are: sodium cromoglycate, a bronchodilator from khellin (*Ammi visnaga*), Metformin, an antidiabetic from galegine (*Galega officinalis*), verapamil a antihypertensive from papaverine (*Papaver somniferum*), aspirin an analgesic from salicin (willow bark), atorvastatin from mevastatin (*Penicillium citrinum*), (**Figure 5**). Malaria remains one of the biggest challenges faced by the mankind, and there is a continuous search for an effective drug. The isolation of quinine from cinchona bark was reported in 1820 by the French pharmacists Caventou and Pelletier. Quinine formed the basis for the synthesis of the commonly used antimalarial drugs. Another antimalarial drug developed from plant lead is artemisinin obtained from *Artemisia annua*. There analogues are used in many countries for the treatment of malaria.

Other noteworthy drugs developed from traditional medicinal plants are: Reserpine an antihypertensive drug from *Rauvolfia serpentina*, Ephedrine from *Ephedra sinica* used as the basis for the synthesis of the anti-asthmatic drug salbutamol and salmeterol, tubocurarine a muscle

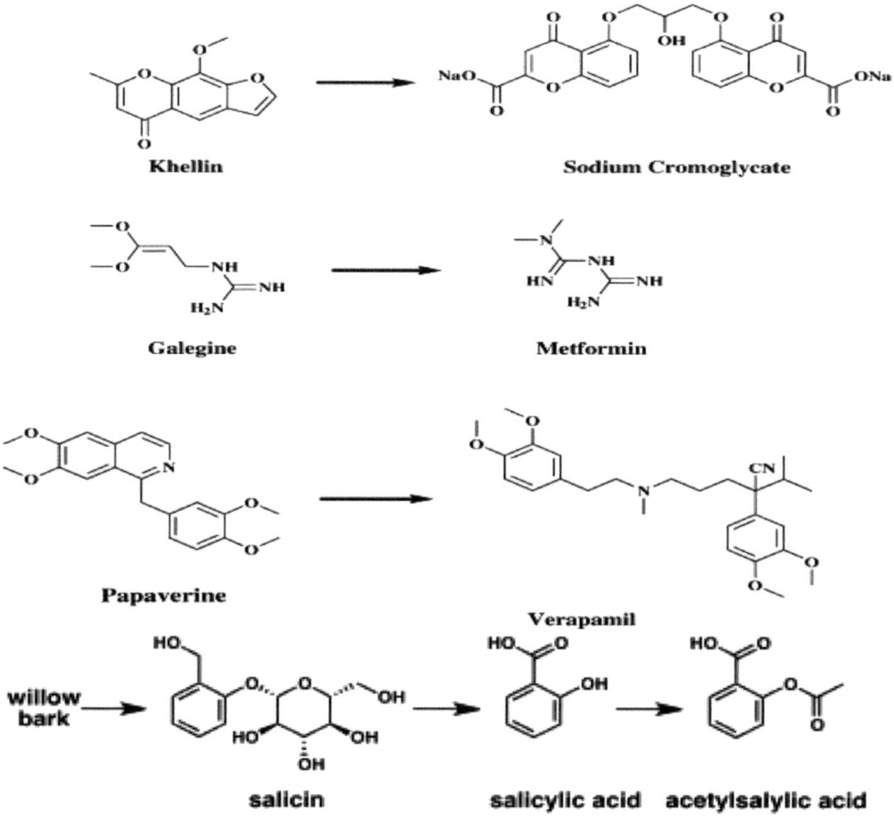

Figure 5. Drugs developed from plant lead molecule.

relaxant, from Curare species. A number of anticancer agents have been obtained from plants: vinblastine and vincristine from *Catharanthus roseus* and two clinically active compounds etoposide and teniposide, Paclitexel most exhilarating anticancer derived from Taxus species. (**Figure 6**).

In addition, recently, various other chemically active agents have gained attention and importantly placed in the arsenal of plant-derived anticancer agents. These are topotecan, irinotecan (CPT-11); belotecan and also their analogues 9-amino and 9-nitro camptochecin. These are semi-synthetic in nature, derived from camptochecin isolated from a Chinese ornamental tree camptotheca acuminate. One of the first plant-derived tubulin interactive compounds recently entered clinical trials, maytansine from the Ethiopian tree *Maytenus serrata*. This plant granted a new lease of life "warhead" (slightly modified), on a monoclonal antibody. The natural product chemists wondered if the compound was microbial in origin due to its similarity to the "ansa" antibiotic such as the rifamycins. Scientists at Takeda during 1977 reported very closely resembled the maytansinoids structure. Thereafter, compounds isolated from bacterium which was renamed as *Actinosynnema pretiosum* in fact similar to those isolated from other plant genera [8].

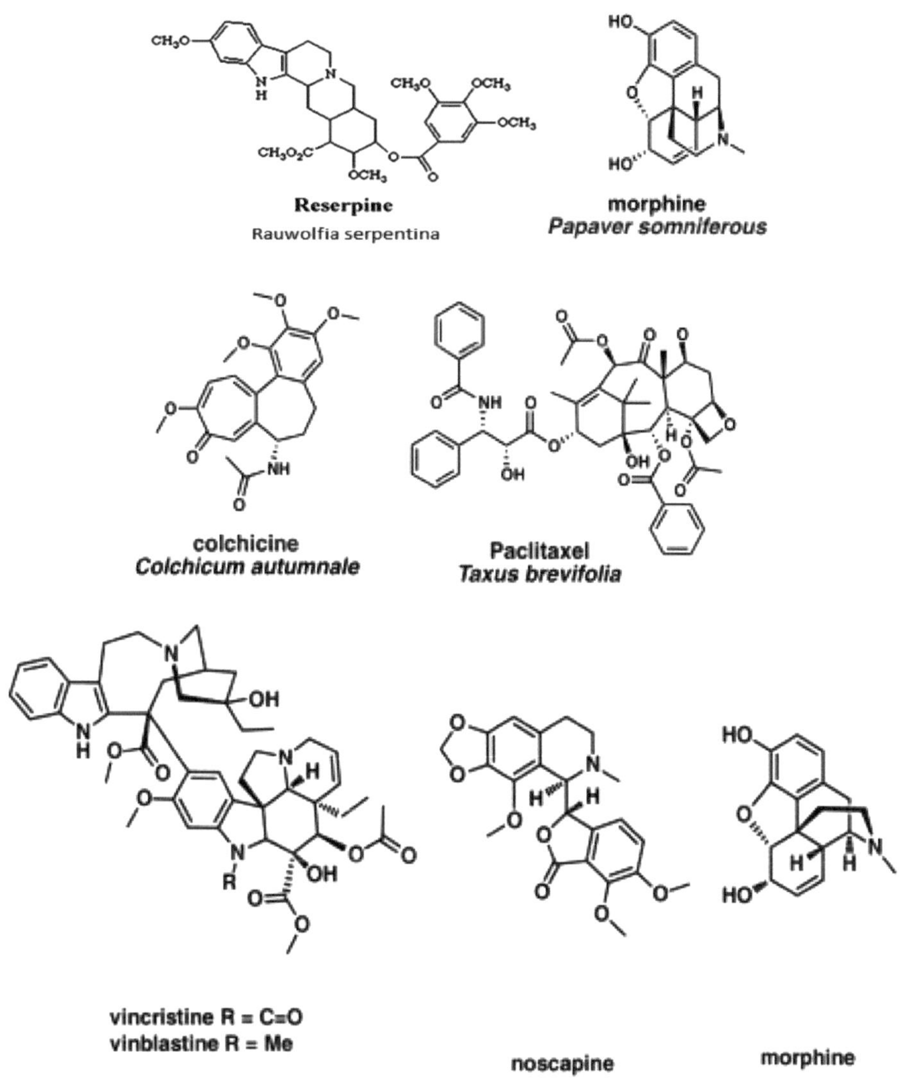

Figure 6. Plant-derived drugs.

2.2. Animals

Amphibians, reptiles and humans have been a fine source of drug. Epibatidine is a potent analgesic obtained from the skin of epipedobates tricolour (A frog). This drug is several times stronger than morphine. But the main snag is that the therapeutic dose of the drug is more close to its toxic dose that drives the development of synthetic analogue. Epibatidine has turned out to be important lead compound for potential novel painkillers. Teprotide isolated from the venom of the snake pit viper, *Bothrops jararaca* led to the design and synthesis of ACE inhibitor Captopril used in the management of hypertension. Another noteworthy finding

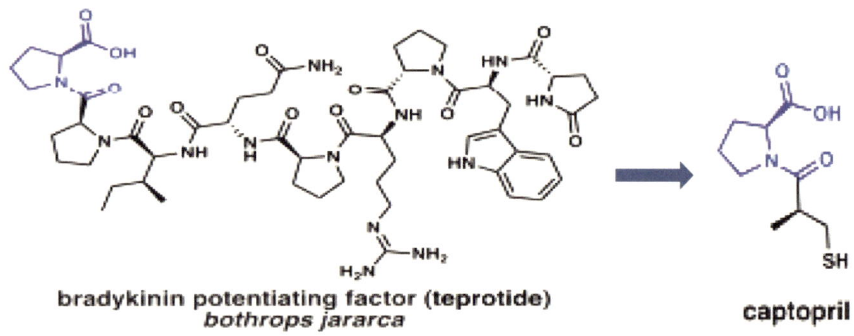

Figure 7. Drug from snake venom.

was the isolation of exendin-4 from the venom of Gila monster, *Heloderma suspectum* that leads to the development of Byetta an injectable antidiabetic drug to control type 2 diabetes. In 2009, a notable peptide having closeness to Human GLP-1 was approved for similar indication in Europe and then in Japan, in 2010, in the USA, under the name liraglutide [9] (**Figure 7**).

2.3. Micro organisms

The discovery of Penicillin from *Penicillium notatum* in 1929 by Fleming steers a new era in medicine "The Golden Era of Antibiotics" and accelerated the investigation of nature for bioactive agents. The microorganisms are the productive source of dissimilar bioactive metabolites and have turned out to be a vital source of drugs in Pharmaceutical industry. These are antibacterial agents: Penicillin from Penicillium species, cephalosporins from *Cephalosporium acremonium*, tetracycline, chloramphenicol, aminoglycosides, rafamycin, and so on. In addition to this immunosuppressive agents like cyclosporins from trichoderma, cholesterol lowering drug such as mevastatin (compactin; from Penicillium species) and lovastatin from Aspergillus species, anthelmintics and antiparasitic drugs like ivermectins from Streptomyces species are all originated from microorganisms [9].

Among the anticancer drugs, anticancer antibiotics plays a significant role in the chemotherapy. These are given in **Table 1**.

2.4. Marine organisms

Seventy five percent of the earth surface has been covered by water, but there is limited research as far as pharmacology of marine organisms is concerned. Many of these are still

S.No.	Anti-tumour antibiotic	Source
1	Bleomycin	Streptomyces verticillus
2	Mitomycin	Streptomyces caespitosus
3	Daunomycin	Streptomyces peucetius
4	Doxorubicin	Streptomyces peucetius var. caesius.

Table 1. Antitumor antibiotics.

unexplored. Marine environment characterises various diverse resources towards new drugs to fight most major diseases like malaria and cancer. Marine environment also signifies an ecological resource consisting of a variety of aquatic plants and animals. Such aquatic organisms are screened for immunomodulatory, antibacterial, antifungal, anti-inflammatory, antimicrobial, neuroprotective, anticancer, analgesic and antimalarial properties. These aquatic organisms are used for new drug developments mostly all over the world. Thus, under the marine pharmacology, there is further scope for research on the drugs of marine origin [10]. Marine pharmacology can be classified on the basis of source of the candidate drug:

- Genetically engineered marine organisms
- Manufacture of pharmaceuticals and nutraceuticals of marine origin
- Chemicals produced by or found in marine organisms shown to have a wide variety of applications as pharmaceuticals.

Classification of marine drugs on the basis of their action (**Table 2**).

Some of the drugs of marine origin approved for human use in different parts of the world are as follows (**Table 3**).

Given underneath are certain marine drugs that are now under Clinical Phase III trial (**Table 4**).

There are some marine drugs that are undergoing Phase II trial (**Table 5**).

Few drugs are also undergoing Clinical Phase I trial (**Table 6**).

Class	Marine drugs
Antibacterial	Eicosapentaenoic acid, isolated from *Phaeodactylum tricornutum* active against gram positive and gram negative bacteria.
Anti-inflammatory	The extracts and other parts of a Mediterranean sponge species *Spongia officinalis* showed anti-inflammatory activity in vivo.
Neuroprotective	Extracts of South Indian green seaweed Ulva reticulate having neuroprotective action.
Antiparasitic	Extracts of Sarcotragus sp. known as Tunisian sponge showed in-vitro anti-leishmanial activity.
Antiviral agents	Exo-polysaccharide extracted from the *Celtodoryx girardae* has Anti-herpes simplex virus-1 (HSV) activity.
Anticancer	Bryostatin, obtained from the Bryozoan, *Bugula neritina*, some forms from sponges and tunicates have cytotoxicity.
Analgesic	Ziconotide, first US FDA approved analgesic of marine origin.
Antimicrobial	The cephalosporins are well-known antimicrobial agents with a marine source of origin.
Antimalarial activity	Isonitrile containing antimalarial molecules have been extracted from the Acanthella sp., a Japanese sponge.

Table 2. Classification of marine drugs.

Approved marine drug	
Cytarabine	It is FDA approved and mainly used in different types of leukaemia, including acute myelocytic leukaemia, lymphocytic leukaemia, meningeal leukaemia, and chronic myelogenous leukaemia.
Vidarabine	It is FDA approved used in recurrent epithelial keratitis caused by HSV type 1 and 2, acute kerato-conjunctivitis, and also for superficial keratitis
Ziconotide	Ziconotide, FDA approved has shown potential as an analgesic.
Trabectedin	A marine product extracted from Ecteinascidia turbinate. First anticancer molecule of marine origin got approval in EU for use in soft-tissue sarcoma and in relapsed cases of platinum-sensitive ovarian cancer

Table 3. Approved drugs of marine origin.

Marine drugs in clinical Phase III trial	
Eribulin mesylate (E7389) or halichondrin B	It is a polyether macrolide natural molecule originally extracted from marine sponges, with potent anticancer activity reported in preclinical animal models. Eribulin is a potent molecule which produces irreversible antimitotic activity leading to cell death by apoptotic pathway.
Soblidotin (auristatin PE or TZT-1027)	Is a synthetic derivative of the dolastatin backbone from dolastatin 10. It is a vascular disrupting agent causing the collapse of the vasculature inside the tumour, in addition to its tubulin inhibitory activity. It is undergoing trials in clinical Phases I, II, and III and companies are trying to use it as a weapon to specific monoclonal antibodies.
Tetrodotoxin	Well-known "marine toxin", and highly substituted guanidine-derivative is not an anti-tumour agent, currently in Phase III trials as analgesic against inadequately controlled pain related to the cancer.

Table 4. Marine drugs in clinical Phase III trial.

Marine drugs in clinical Phase II trial	
DMXBA (GTS-21) [3-(2,4-dimethoxybenzylidene) -anabaseine; GTS-21]	It is a synthetic imitative of anabaseine, an alkaloid found in many species of aquatic worms of phylum nemertea. It is reported to be beneficial for improving cognition and sensory gating deficiency in a variety of laboratory animals.
Plitidepsin	It is a natural marine depsipeptide, currently obtained by total synthesis. It was primarily isolated from a tunicate *Aplidium albicans* found in the Mediterranean Sea. It is a highly potent apoptosis inducer.
Elisidepsin (PM02734)	It is a novel cyclic peptide derived from marine sources belonging to the Kahalalide family. It is now in Phase II with proof of antitumor potency with positive therapeutic index.
PM00104 (Zalypsis)	It is linked to jorumycin extracted from the Pacific nudibranch's (*Jorunna funebris*) skin and mucus as well as from renieramiycins extracted from varieties of sponges and tunicates. Preclinical in vivo studies indicated high antitumor activity in cells of breast, prostate and renal cancers with a modest antitumor action on colon cancer cells.
Plinabulin (NPI-2358)	It is a fully laboratory made analog of the natural product halimide originally derived from marine Aspergillus sp. CNC-139 and phenylahistin extracted from Aspergillus ustus. It inhibits the polymerisation of tubulin, resulting in destabilisation of the vascular endothelial cells of the tumour.

Marine drugs in clinical Phase II trial	
ILX-651 (tasidotin or synthadotin)	A synthetic derivative of dolastatin-15 and it inhibits assembly of tubulin. It is an orally active drug and has progressed to Phase II trials in different types of cancer.
Pseudopterosins	A leading class of diterpene glycosides primarily extracted from the octocoral *Pseudopterogorgia elisabethae*. It is a strong phorbol myristate acetate inhibitor. In a double-blind, Phase II clinical trial, the drug was found to augment re-epithelialisation process in early wound repair process.

Table 5. Marine drugs in clinical Phase II trial.

Marine drugs in clinical Phase I trial	
Leconotide (AM-336, ω-conotoxin CVID)	It is a peptide similar to Ziconotide and is undergoing Phase I trials for the treatment of cancer.
Enfortumab vedotin	It is used in immunotherapy, and it is a combination of a fully human IgG1k antibody and monomethyl auristatin E.
Vorsetuzumab mafdotin (SGN-75)	An antibody-drug conjugate, with monomethyl-auristatin F attached to the anti-CD70 monoclonal humanised antibody 1F6. This molecule is presently being evaluated for its value in relapsed and refractory non-Hodgkin's lymphoma in Phase I clinical trials and also in metastatic renal cancer.

Table 6. Marine drugs in clinical Phase I trial.

3. Natural product drug discovery and development: an integrative approach

An integrative approach comprising various discovery tools and novel discipline would definitely endow with an input in natural product drug discovery and development. Natural product can be envisaged to remain an indispensable component in the development of new drug. According to Lutz natural product not only complement synthetic molecule, they also exhibit drug-related features unsurpassable by any synthetic compound. An important attribute of natural product is their huge structure and chemical diversity. Another beneficial feature of natural product is their biological history. The natural products possess an inherent ability to interact with other molecules, which is a crucial precondition for making a drug. The natural product due to its sterically more complex structure exhibit advanced binding properly compared with synthetics. The natural products are perceived as "drug like-ness" and "biological friendliness" than totally synthetic molecule making them apposite lead candidates.

The process of drug discovery involves the identification of candidates, synthesis, screening, characterisation and assays for therapeutic efficacy, which in fact is a very lengthy and tedious process. Considering the success of natural products as source of new drugs, new technologies have emerged to facilitate the process. These technologies are combinatorial chemistry, high throughput screening (HTS), bioinformatics, proteomics and genomics.

Other recently developed techniques are molecular diversity, compound library design, MMR based screening, QSAR and computer-aided drug design.

3.1. Combinatorial chemistry

Combinatorial chemistry involves the rapid synthesis or the computer simulation of a large number of different but often structurally related molecules or materials. In a combinatorial synthesis, the number of compounds made increases exponentially with the number of chemical steps. In a binary light-directed synthesis, 2n compounds can be made in n chemical steps. Combinatorial chemistry is especially common in computer aided drug design (CADD) and can be done online with web-based software, such as mole inspiration.

3.1.1. Principle of combinatorial chemistry

Combinatorial chemistry is a technique by which large numbers of structurally distinct molecules may be synthesised in a time and submitted for pharmacological assay. The key of combinatorial chemistry is that a large range of analogues is synthesised using the same reaction conditions, the same reaction vessels. In this way, the chemist can synthesise many hundreds or thousands of compounds in one time instead of preparing only a few by simple methodology.

The conventional approach of synthesis is

$$A + B \rightarrow AB$$

In contrast to this approach, combinatorial chemistry offer the potential to make every combination of compound A1 to An with compound B1 to Bn.

Compound Libraries $\xrightarrow{\textbf{Screening}}$ **Lead Compounds** $\xleftrightarrow{\textbf{Optimization}}$ **In -Vivo Studies**

The range of combinatorial techniques is highly diverse, and these products could be made individually in a parallel or in mixtures, using either solution or solid phase techniques.

Combinatorial Chemistry is used to synthesise large number of chemical compounds by combining sets of building blocks. Each newly synthesised compound's composition is slightly different from the previous one. A traditional chemist can synthesise 100–200 compounds per year. A combinatorial robotic system can produce in a year thousands or millions compounds, which can be tested for potential drug candidates in a high-throughput screening process [11].

3.2. High throughput screening

High throughput screening is a standard method for hit discovery for scientific experimentation in drug discovery and allied field. HTS uses robotics, data processing and control software, liquid handling devices and sensitive detectors making researchers to quickly conduct the biochemical, genetic or pharmacological tests. Employing HTS, it is comparatively trouble-free and swift to identify active compounds. HTS is hassle free technique that collects large amount of experimental data in a relatively short time [11].

3.3. Bioinformatics, proteomics and genomics

Genomics and proteomics in combination with combinatorial chemistry and high-throughput screening are helping to bring forward an unparalleled number of potential lead compounds. Proteomics includes technologies for protein mapping that is separating, distinguishing and quantifying the proteins in samples and also identification and characterisation of specific protein. The main protein mapping technology currently in use is two-dimensional polyacrylamide gel electrophoresis (2D-PAGE) that can resolve up to 2000 proteins in single gel.

Genomics is an area within genetics that concerns the sequencing and analysis of an organism's genome. The genome is the entire DNA content that is present within one cell of an organism. Experts in genomics strive to determine complete DNA sequences and perform genetic mapping to help understand disease. Since many diseases occurs due to failure of genes to perform correctly, genomics help to identify the genes involved in responsiveness to a given drug. Hence, genomics is an integral part of drug discovery [12].

4. Challenges with natural products

In spite of so many inherent advantages of these natural products for the synthesis of various molecules ranging from simple skeleton to highly complex chemical structures, they do have certain potential limitations.

- Drug discovery from natural products would eventually lead to its commercialisation. This may further burden the natural resource and consequently lead to undesirable environmental concerns. While synthesis of active molecule could be an option, not every molecule is amenable for complete synthesis. Hence, certain degree of dependence on lead resource would continue, for example, anticancer agent like etoposide, docetaxel, paclitaxel. It is expected that around 25,000 plant species would cease to exit by the end of this century.
- Another issue, the IPR protection related to the natural products is creating some confusion because the lead compounds are based on some linkage to traditional uses.

These processes impede the pace of discovery process at various levels. Challenges in the new drug developments are mainly due to:

i. Existing prototype for drug discovery in large pharmaceutical industries.

ii. Technical limitation of natural products

According to Koehn and Carter, the unique feature/characters of the compound isolated from natural products are:

a. Increased steric complexity

b. Presence of large number chiral centres

c. Presence of greater number of oxygen atoms

d. Ratio of aromatic ring atoms to total heavy atoms, that is, low

e. Molecular rigidity is high

f. Wider distribution of molecular properties, such as molecular mass, O/w partition coefficient and diversity of ring system [13].

It is presumed that large number of NP despite being biologically active and having favourable pharmacokinetic profile do not satisfy the criteria "drug likeness." The challenge is of building a physio-chemical tuned natural products library in line c the lead generation to promote natural products to their full potential. Therefore, ultimately, the biggest challenge is to find alternative drug ability criteria for the compound of natural origin, as they do not fit "rule of five" for to be drug like. As per rule of five propagated by Lipinski [14], a drug candidate should have:

i. Less than 10 H bond acceptors

ii. Less than 5 H bond acceptors

iii. Mol, wet >500 Da

iv. PK of less than 5

5. Conclusion

Natural product drug discovery, ethno-pharmacology, traditional and attractive medicines are re-emerging as new strategic options. The chapter endeavoured that novel-natural products can be optimised on the basis of their biological activities using highly sophisticated combinatorial biosynthetic techniques, microbial genomes and screening process.

The chapter made efforts to provide short-lived imprint of the significance of natural products as bioactive molecules and also as pharmaceutical agents. On the advent of novel screening systems related to the discovery of genetic information accelerating the need to rapidly identify effective and novel lead structures as important necessity. It is certain that an important portion of these leads will remain to be resultant natural product.

As on today, comparative ease of access to plants now resulted in the discovery of a plant-derived compounds, so far as the microbial sources are particularly important in the area of antibiotic. Further effort suggests, that marine organisms, and such group of organisms not much published, the marine-sourced fungi shall perform progressively significant role in the future. This role especially when given the impressive advances in the power of organic synthesis to report the supply problems intrinsic with this source material. With the arrival of genetic techniques that permit the isolation and expression of biosynthetic cases in the future, microbes and their marine invertebrate hosts might better be the new frontier towards natural products lead discovery. Plant endophytes also offer stimulating new resource.

Forthcoming features of antibiotic discovery and development include somewhat from a different perspective, a significant number of issues referred to in this chapter. Together with these novel sources to refurbished phenotypic screens that employ high-content imaging systems and that can run in microliter volumes, it might enable investigators to speedily evaluate the activity of individual agents and their potential.

Author details

Seema Kohli

Address all correspondence to: seemankohli@gmail.com

Pharmacy Department, K.N. Polytechnic College Jabalpur, Madhya Pradesh, India

References

[1] Lahlou M. The success of natural products in drug discovery. Pharmacology and Pharmacy. 2013;**4**:17-31

[2] Famsworth NR, Akerele O, Bingel AS, Soejarto DD, Guo Z. Medicinal plants in therapy. Bulletin of the World Health Organisation. 1985;**63**:965-981

[3] Ulrich-Merzenich G, Panek D, Zeiltor H, Velter H, Wagnes H. Drug development from natural products: Expoliting synergistic effects, Indian. The Journal of Experimental Biology. 2010;**48**:208-219

[4] Pawar HA. Natural product as a source of lead to the design of new drugs. Natural Products Chemistry & Research. 2014;**2**(6):156. DOI: 10.4172/2329-6836.1000156

[5] Cragg GM, Newman DJ. Biodiversity: A continuing source of novel drug leads. Pure and Applied Chemistry. 2005;**77**(1):7-24

[6] Patwardhan B, Vaidya ADB. Natural products drug discovery: Accelerating the clinical candidate development using reverse pharmacology approaches, Indian. The Journal of Experimental Biology. 2010;**48**:220-227

[7] Bhutani KK, Gohil VSM. Natural products drug discovery research in India: Status and appraisal. Indian Journal of Experimental Biology. 2010;**48**:199-207

[8] Balunas MJ, Douglas Kinghorn A. Drug discovery from medicinal plants. Life Sciences. 2005;**78**:431-441

[9] Cragg GM, Newman DJ. Natural products: A continue source of novel drug leads. Biochemica et Biophysica Acta. 2013;**1830**:3670-3695

[10] Malve H. Exploring the ocean for new drug developments marin pharmacology. Journal of Pharmacy & Bioallied Sciences. 2016;**8**(2):83-91

[11] Rasheed A, Farhat R. Cominatorial Chemistry: A Review. International Journal of Pharmaceutical Sciences and Research. 2013;**4**(7):2502-2516

[12] Sharma N, Harikumar SL. Use of genomics and proteomics in pharmaceutical drug discovery and development. International Journal of Pharmacy and Pharmaceutical Sciences. 2013;**3**(15):975-1491

[13] Katiyar C. Drug discovery from plant sources: An integrated approach. An International Quarterly Journal of Research in Ayurveda. 2015;**33**(1):10-19

[14] Lipinski CA, Lombardo F, Dominy BW, Feeney PJ. Experimental and computational approaches to estimates solubility and permeability in drug discovery and development settings. Advanced Drug Delivery Reviews. 2001;**46**:3-26

Section 2

Specific Molecular Mechanism and Lead Compounds for Drug Design

Chapter 4

Molecular Classification of Antitubulin Agents with Indole Ring Binding at Colchicine-Binding Site

Francisco Torrens and Gloria Castellano

Additional information is available at the end of the chapter

http://dx.doi.org/10.5772/intechopen.73744

Abstract

Algorithms for classification and taxonomy are proposed based on criteria as *information entropy* and its production. A set of 59 antitubulin agents with trimethoxyphenyl (TMP), indole, and C=O bridge present inhibition of gastric cancer cell line MNK-45. On the basis of structure-activity relation of TMPs, derivatives are designed that are classified using seven structural parameters of different moieties. A lot of categorization methods are founded on the entropy of information. On using processes on collections of reasonable dimension, an extreme amount of outcomes occur, matching information and suffering a combinatorial increase. Notwithstanding, following the *equipartition conjecture*, an assortment factor appears among dissimilar alternatives resultant from categorization among pecking order rankings. The entropy of information allows classifying the compounds and agrees with principal component analyses. A table of periodic properties TMPs is obtained. Features denote positions R_{1-4} on the benzo and $X-R_{5/6}$ on the pyridine ring in indole cycle. Inhibitors in the same group are suggested to present similar properties; those in the same group and period will present maximum resemblance.

Keywords: periodic law, periodic property, periodic table, information entropy, equipartition conjecture, anticancer activity

1. Introduction

Experimentally, antitubulin analogues were synthesized/tested for antitubulin activity, revealing ligand-interaction principles with tubulin/related bioactivity [1–13]. Molecular modeling studies of antitubulin agents were performed to aid in the design of better antitubulin inhibitors [14–16]. In computer-aided drug design studies, comparative molecular field analysis

(CoMFA) combined with docking calculations was applied to protein-ligand-binding complexes [17–21]. A class of antitubulin agents, binding at colchicine (COL) site with an indole ring, was developed and underwent examinations for binding, antitubulin polymerization, and/or anticancer effects. The discovered properties are helpful for better-inhibitor design. Half inhibitory concentrations (IC_{50}) were collected for the inhibition of gastric cancer cell MKN-45, for 59 COL-like compounds with indole and trimethoxyphenyl (TMP) rings (**Figure 1**), which bind at COL site [22]. The IC_{50} were measured for 24 compounds and reviewed for others: 71 compounds were collected. Trial CoMFA calculations for all gave a low leave-one-out determination coefficient q^2~0.2. Examination of functional groups showed that three ones are much more bulky than the others. Functional groups of eight are much different from others. Compounds were excluded leaving 59 substances in CoMFA calculation. With data, three-dimensional (3D)-quantitative structure-activity relationship (SAR) (QSAR) examination was performed with CoMFA [23], combined with docking calculations for compounds to illustrate correlation of functional group variations with anticancer effect. An approach was employed to examine QSAR for a number of other protein-ligand-binding complexes. Functional-group substitutions locate at sites around indole ring, i.e., $R_{1–6}$ functional-group sites. Comparative QSAR modeling of 2-phenylindole-3-carbaldehyde derivatives was performed as potential antimitotic agents [24]. The KIT kinase mutants showed unique mechanisms of drug resistance to imatinib and sunitinib in gastrointestinal stromal tumor patients [25]. Gene expression profiling of gastric cancer was reported [26]. Natural product COL, obtained from *Colchicum autumnale*, is a bioactive alkaloid used in the treatment of a number of diseases [27]. It received considerable attention in the basic study of neoplasia by its capacity for interrupting *mitosis*, ending the process in metaphase [28]. The COL acts as an inhibitor of the polymerization of tubulin (a protein that contains eight Trp units) [29]. It was used as a probe to understand *microtubule* role in cells because of its big affinity to tubulin, in which structure presents a binding site (*colchicine domain*) [30, 31]. Tubulin is a target for cancer treatment: a number of drugs were developed to target it [32]. Binding with it, ligands interfere with its polymerization dynamics and exhibit an antitumor effect. In addition to developed drugs (*viz.* taxol, vibrestine), which bind with it at taxol/vibrestine-binding sites, COL presents a tubulin binding site and showed anticancer effects although with significant toxicity. Developing COL-like compounds with lesser toxicity represented an effort in finding better ligands to target tubulin at COL-binding site [33, 34]. A simple computerized algorithm useful for establishing a relation

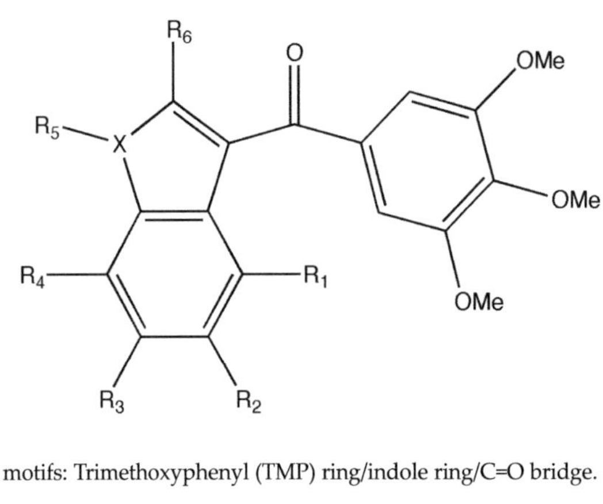

Figure 1. General structure motifs: Trimethoxyphenyl (TMP) ring/indole ring/C=O bridge.

between chemical structures [35, 36] was proposed. The preliminary idea results the entropy of information for configuration detection. The entropy of information results was expressed based on a *similarity matrix* among a pair of chemical entities. Because the entropy of information results feebly discerning for categorization reasons, the more influential concepts of *entropy production* and *equipartition conjecture* result were presented in [37]. In previous articles, the classifications by periodic properties of local anesthetics [38–40], inhibitors of human immunodeficiency virus [41–43], and anticancer drugs [44, 45] were analyzed. The goal of the current account is expanding the promises of knowledge of the algorithm and, as compounds are unaffectedly explained by a changeable-dimension prearranged model, learning universal methods in the dispensation of prearranged information. Next goal presents a periodic classification of TMPs. A further objective is to perform a validation of the periodic table (PT) with an external property not used in the development of PT.

2. Computational method

The key problem in classification studies is to define *similarity indices* when several criteria of comparison are involved. The primary stage in counting resemblance for TMPs records the majority of the significant moieties. The *vector of properties* $\bar{i} = \langle i_1, i_2, \ldots i_k, \ldots \rangle$ should be linked to each TMP *i*, whose parts match with dissimilar characteristic groups in the molecule, in a pecking order consistent the predictable significance of pharmacological potency. Whether moiety *m-th* results more important than portion *k-th* then $m < k$. The parts i_k are values "1" or "0", consistent if an alike portion of rank *k* is present in TMP *i* contrasted to the recommendation one. The examination comprises two regions of structure variation in TMP molecules: positions $R_{1–4}$ on the benzo and locations X and $R_{5/6}$ on the pyridine ring in the indole cycle. The TMPs are inhibitory to gastric cancer cell line MKN-45. The *structural elements* of a TMP molecule can be *ranked* according to their contribution to MKN-45 inhibition in the order: $R_1 > R_4 > R_2 > X > R_5 > R_3 > R_6$. Index $i_1 = 1$ denotes R_1 = H ($i_1 = 0$, otherwise), $i_2 = 1$ means R_4 = H, $i_3 = 1$ signifies R_2 = H, $i_4 = 1$ stands for X = N, $i_5 = 1$ indicates R_5 = H, $i_6 = 1$ represents R_3 = OMe, and $i_7 = 1$ implies $R_6 = CH_2–OH$. In TMP 42, $R_1 = R_4 = R_2 = R_5$ = H, X = N, R_3 = OMe and $R_6 = CH_2–OH$; obviously its associated vector is <1,111,111>. The TMP 42 was selected as *reference* because of its greatest MNK-45 inhibition. Vectors were associated with 59 TMPs with gastric anticancer activities. Vector <1,111,110> is associated with TMP 1 since $R_1 = R_4 = R_2 = R_5 = R_6$ = H, X = N and R_3 = OMe. Mean by r_{ij} ($0 \le r_{ij} \le 1$) the similarity index of a pair of TMPs linked to vectors $\bar{i}$ and $\bar{j}$, in that order. The relationship of similarity results is typified by a *similarity matrix* $\mathbf{R} = [r_{ij}]$. The similarity index among a pair of TMPs $\bar{i} = \langle i_1, i_2, \ldots i_k \ldots \rangle$ and $\bar{j} = \langle j_1, j_2, \ldots j_k \ldots \rangle$ is described by:

$$r_{ij} = \sum_k t_k (a_k)^k \quad (k = 1, 2, \ldots) \tag{1}$$

where $0 \le a_k \le 1$ and $t_k = 1$ whether $i_k = j_k$ except $t_k = 0$ whether $i_k \neq j_k$. The definition allocates a weight $(a_k)^k$ to whichever feature concerned about the explanation of molecule *i* or *j*. The MNK-45 gastric cancer inhibition data reported by Lin *et al.* were used for the present classification study. The *grouping algorithm* applies the *stabilized* similarity matrix obtained *via* the *max-min composition rule o* as described by:

$$(\mathbf{RoS})_{ij} = \max_k\left[\min_k\left(r_{ik}, s_{kj}\right)\right] \tag{2}$$

where $\mathbf{R} = [r_{ij}]$ and $\mathbf{S} = [s_{ij}]$ that result in matrices of the same kind and $(\mathbf{RoS})_{ij}$, entry (i,j)*-th* of matrix **RoS** [46–49]. On using composition rule max-min iteratively, so that $\mathbf{R}(n + 1) = \mathbf{R}(n)$ o $\mathbf{R}$, an integer n results fulfilling: $\mathbf{R}(n) = \mathbf{R}(n + 1) = \ldots$ The resultant matrix $\mathbf{R}(n)$ is named as *stabilized similarity matrix*. The importance of stabilization stretches out in the categorization procedure, and stabilization generates a separation in displaced divisions. From the present on, it results implicitly that the stabilized similarity matrix is applied and named as $\mathbf{R}(n) = [r_{ij}(n)]$. The *grouping rule* is as follows: i and j results allocated in the same division whether $r_{ij}(n) \geq b$. The grouping of i ($\widehat{i}$) results in the collection of molecules j that fulfills the grouping rule $r_{ij}(n) \geq b$. The matrix of clusters results in

$$\widehat{\mathbf{R}}\,(n) = \left[\widehat{r}_{\widehat{i}\,\widehat{j}}\right] = \max_{s,\,t}(r_{st}) \quad \left(s \in \widehat{i}, t \in \widehat{j}\right) \tag{3}$$

where s means whichever indicator of a molecule fitting in class $\widehat{i}$ (likewise for t and $\widehat{j}$). Rule (3) denotes discovering the main similarity index among molecules of a pair of divisions. In information theory, *information entropy h* measures the surprise that the source emitting the sequences can give [50, 51]. We consider the utilization of a qualitative mark assay to decide the attendance of Fe in a sample of water. With no sample in the past, the analyst has to start with the pair of results supposing: 0 (Fe not present) and 1 (Fe there), which are equiprobable with likelihood 1/2. As up to a pair of elements are there in the sample solution (e.g., Fe, Ni or both), there are four achievable results neither from (0, 0) to the two being there (1, 1) *via* on a par likelihood $1/2^2$. Which of the four options goes is decided by a pair of assays, each one with a pair of clear conditions. Likewise, with three metals, there are eight options, every one with a likelihood $1/2^3$: three assays are necessary. The following configuration clearly connects uncertainty to information necessary to solve it. The amount of options results stated to the power of 2. The power to which 2 is lifted to provide the amount of occurrences N results in the logarithm to base 2 of that amount. Both information and uncertainty are described in terms of the logarithm to base 2 of the amount of achievable analytical results: $\log_2 N$. The initial uncertainty is defined in terms of the probability of the occurrence of every outcome; e.g., the definition is as follows: $I = H = \log_2 N = \log_2 1/p = -\log_2 p$, where I denotes the information held in the reply provided that there were N options, H, the first uncertainty coming from the necessity of taking into account the N options and p, the likelihood of each result whether or not all N occurrences are evenly probable to occur. The equation can be extended to the case in which the likelihood of each result does not result the same; whether it is identified from historical experiment is proven by some metals that result in more probability than other ones, the expression results are corrected so that the logarithms of the particular likelihood appropriately weighted result in: $H = -\Sigma\, p_i \log_2 p_i$, where: $\Sigma\, p_i = 1$. Take into account the first case but at present, historical experiment proved that 90% of the samples had no Fe. The amount of uncertainty results is computed as: $H = -(0.9 \log_2 0.9 + 0.1 \log_2 0.1) = 0.469$ bits. For a particular case happening with probability p, the amount of astonishment results is proportional to –ln p. Extending the outcome to a random variable X (that is able to present N achievable values x_1, …, x_N with probabilities p_1, …, p_N), the astonishing mean is obtained when finding out the value of X results $-\Sigma\, p_i \ln p_i$. The entropy of information is linked to similarity matrix **R** results:

$$h(\mathbf{R}) = -\sum_{i,j} r_{ij}\ln r_{ij} - \sum_{i,j} (1 - r_{ij})\ln(1 - r_{ij}) \tag{4}$$

Mean is obtained by C_b, the collection of divisions and $\widehat{\mathbf{R}}_b$, the similarity matrix at the classification level b. The entropy of information fulfills the following features. (1) $h(\mathbf{R}) = 0$ whether $r_{ij} = 0$ or $r_{ij} = 1$. (2) $h(\mathbf{R})$ results maximum whether $r_{ij} = 0.5$, i.e., as the ambiguity is maximum. (3) $h\left(\widehat{\mathbf{R}}_b\right) \le h(\mathbf{R})$ for whichever b, i.e., categorization directs to a deficit of entropy. (4) $h\left(\widehat{\mathbf{R}}_{b_1}\right) \le h\left(\widehat{\mathbf{R}}_{b_2}\right)$ if $b_1 < b_2$, i.e., entropy is a monotone function of grouping level b. In the categorization procedure, each *hierarchical tree* matches to a reliance of the entropy of information on the classification level, and a plot h–b is obtained. The *equipartition conjecture of entropy production* of Tondeur and Kvaalen results is suggested as an assortment principle, between dissimilar alternatives coming from categorization between pecking order rankings. Consistent with the conjecture, for a provided custody, the top arrangement of a dendrogram results in which the production of entropy results is mainly dispersed regularly, i.e., neighboring a type of equipartition. It is gone on at this point similarly *via information entropy* in its place of thermodynamic entropy. Equipartition entails a linear relationship, i.e., a steady production of entropy of information all along the extent of b, so that the *equipartition line* results are explained by:

$$h_{\text{eqp}} = h_{\max} b \tag{5}$$

As the categorization results are disconnected, a mean of stating equipartition is a usual staircase function. The most excellent alternative results decided the one minimizing the addition of the square differences:

$$SS = \sum_{b_i} \left(h - h_{\text{eqp}}\right)^2 \tag{6}$$

Learning procedures alike the ones met in *stochastic methods* are the results as applied in [52]. Taking into account a provided classification as *good* or perfect from practice or experience, which matches to a *reference* similarity matrix $\mathbf{S} = [s_{ij}]$ obtained for equivalent weights $a_1 = a_2 = \ldots = a$ and any amount of fabricated features. Then, take into account identical collection of molecules as in the good categorization and the real features. The similarity index r_{ij} results calculated with Eq. (1) provided matrix **R**. The amount of features for **R** and **S** can vary. The learning process lies in attempting to get categorization outcomes for **R** as near as likely to the *good* categorization. The primary weight a_1 results obtained constant and just the next weights a_2, a_3,... result exposed to random changes. A novel similarity matrix results *via* Eq. (1) and the novel weights. The distance among the classifications typified by **R** and **S** results is provided by:

$$D = -\sum_{ij}(1 - r_{ij})\ln\frac{1 - r_{ij}}{1 - s_{ij}} - \sum_{ij} r_{ij}\ln\frac{r_{ij}}{s_{ij}} \quad \forall 0 \leq r_{ij}, s_{ij} \leq 1 \tag{7}$$

The definition was suggested by Kullback to measure the distance between two probability distributions, which is an amount of the distance among matrices **R** and **S** [53]. As for each matrix a matching categorization exists, the pair of categorizations result contrasted by distance, which results a non-negative amount that approximates zero as the similarity among **R** and **S** rises. The outcome of the procedure results a collection of weights permitting proper categorization. The algorithm was utilized in the production of complicated dendrograms *via* the entropy of information [54]. Our program MolClas is an easy, dependable, effective, and quick process for molecular categorization, founded on the conjecture of the equipartition of the production of the entropy of information consistent with Eqs. (1)–(7). It reads the amount of features and molecular indices. It permits the optimization of the coefficients. It not obligatorily reads the initial coefficients and the amount of iteration cycles. The correlation matrix results are computed by the algorithm or read from input. Code MolClas permits the alteration of the correlation matrix from [−1, 1] to [0, 1]. The program computes the similarity matrix of the features in symmetric storage mode, computes categorizations, checks whether categorizations result is dissimilar, computes distances among categorizations, computes the similarity matrices of categorizations, works out the entropy of information of categorizations, optimizes coefficients, carries out single/complete-linkage hierarchical cluster analyses, and charts classification plots. It was written not only to analyze the equipartition conjecture of entropy production but also to explore the world of molecular classification. Code MolClas is different from other program MolClass as referred in the literature [55]. While MolClas classifies molecules based on hierarchical dichotomic (Boolean) descriptors, MolClass discovers SARs from molecular patterns (*fingerprints*) extracted from experimental datasets and needs to interrogate big databases (PubChem, ChEMBL, ChemBank). Code MolClas is available at Internet (torrens@uv.es) and is free for academic use.

3. Calculation results and discussion

Matrix of Pearson correlation coefficients results computed among couples of vector properties $<i_1,i_2,i_3,i_4,i_5,i_6,i_7>$ for 59 TMPs. Pearson correlations result displayed in the partial correlation diagram, which encloses high ($r \geq 0.75$), medium ($0.50 \leq r < 0.75$), low ($0.25 \leq r < 0.50$), and *zero* ($r < 0.25$) partial correlations. Couples of inhibitors with superior partial associations present a vector property alike. Notwithstanding, the outcomes have to be gotten with concern since the TMP with steady vector <1,111,111> (Entry 42) presents zero standard deviation, producing

http://dx.doi.org/10.5772/intechopen.73744

maximum partial correlation $r = 1$ with whichever TMP, which results an artifact. After the conjecture of equipartition, the intercorrelations are illustrated in the partial correlation diagram, which contains 1382 high (**Figure 2**, *red lines*), 109 medium (*orange*), 161 low (*yellow*), and 59 *zero* (*black*) partial correlations. Six out of 58 high partial correlations of Entry 42 were corrected; e.g., its correlations with Entries 3 and 47 are medium, its correlations with Entries 12, 15, and 43 are low, and its correlation with Entry 46 is *zero* partial correlation.

The grouping rule in the case with equal weights $a_k = 0.5$ for $b_1 = 0.97$ allows the classes:

C–b_1 = (1,5–8,10,11,13,16,17,26–28,41,42,44,45,48,58,59),(2,4,9,18,19,49),(3),(12),

(14,20–25,29–33,35,50–55),(15,43),(34,36–40,56,57),(46),(47)

The nine groupings are obtained with associated entropy h–**R**–b_1 = 39.44. The *dendrogram* (binary tree) matching with <$i_1,i_2,i_3,i_4,i_5,i_6,i_7$ > and C–b_1 is calculated [56–58]; it provides a binary taxonomy that separates the same nine classes: from top to bottom, the data bifurcate into groupings 3, 4, 8, 9, 1, 2, 5, 6, and 7 with 1, 1, 1, 1, 20, 6, 19, 2, and 8 TMPs, respectively [59]. The TMPs 42, 26, etc. with the greatest inhibitory activity are grouped into the same class.

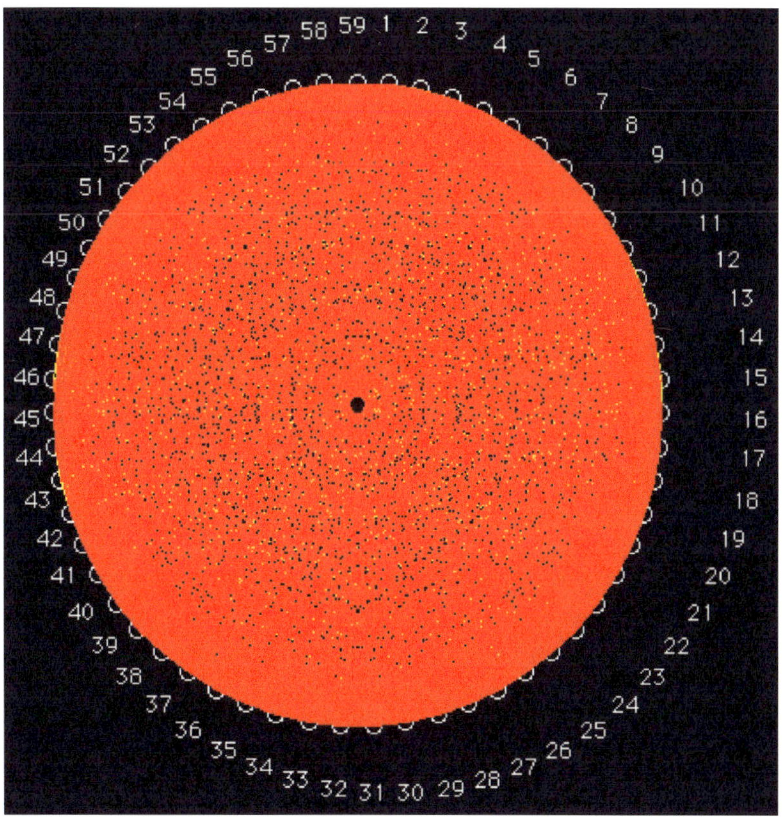

Figure 2. Partial correlation diagram: High (*red*), medium (*orange*), and low (*yellow*) correlations.

The TMPs in the same grouping appear highly correlated in the partial correlation diagram. At level b_2 with $b_2 = 0.86$, the set of classes results in:

C–b_2 = (1,4–8,10,11,13,14,16–42,44,45,48–59),(2,9),(3,47),(12,15),(43),(46).

Six classes result and entropy decays to h–**R**–b_2 = 16.18. Dendrogram matching to $<i_1,i_2,i_3,i_4,i_5,i_6,i_7>$ and C–b_2 divides the same six classes: from top to bottom data bifurcate into classes 5, 6, 1, 2, 3, and 4 with 1, 1, 51, 2, 2, and 2 TMPs, respectively. Again, TMPs with the greatest inhibitory potency belong to the same class. The TMPs in the same class appear highly correlated in the partial correlation diagram and dendrogram. An analysis of set containing 1–59 classes was performed, in agreement with partial correlation diagram and dendrograms. In view of partial correlation diagram and dendrograms, we split data into seven classes: (1,26–28,41,42,45,58,59), (5–8,10,11,13,16,17,44,48), (14,20–25,29–33,35,50–55), (34,36–40,56,57), (2,4,9,18,19,49), (3,47), and (12,15,43,46). **Figure 3** displays corresponding tree. Again, TMPs with the greatest activity correspond to the same class.

The illustration of the classification above in a radial tree (**Figure 4**) shows the same classes, in qualitative agreement with the partial correlation diagram and dendrograms. Once more, TMPs with the greatest potency are included in the same grouping.

Program SplitsTree analyzes cluster analysis (CA) data [60]. Based on *split decomposition*, it takes a *distance matrix* and produces a graph that represents the relations between taxa. For ideal data, graph is a tree, whereas less ideal data cause a tree-like network, which is interpreted as possible evidence for different and conflicting data. As split decomposition does not attempt to force data on to a tree, it gives a good indication of how *tree*-like are given data. Splits graph for 59 TMPs in (**Figure 5**) shows that most TMP groups collapse: (1,2,4–11,13,16–19,26–28,41,42,44,45,48,49,58,59), (3,47), (12,15,43), (14,20–25,29–33,35,50–55), and (34,36–40,56,57); classes 1, 2, and 5 coincide. No conflicting relation appears between TMPs. Splits graph is in partial agreement with partial correlation diagram, dendrograms, and radial tree.

Usually in quantitative structure-property relationships (QSPRs), the information archive encloses fewer than 100 molecules and thousands of X-variables. There are a lot of X-variables that nobody is able to find out by *inspection* configurations, tendencies, groupings, etc. in the molecules. *Principal component analysis* (PCA) results a method helpful to *summarize* the knowledge enclosed in the **X**-matrix and place it comprehensible [61–66]. The PCA acts by decomposing the **X**-matrix as the product of two matrices **P** and **T**. The *loading matrix* (**P**), with knowledge concerning the variables, encloses some vectors [*principal components* (PCs)], in which results are obtained as linear combinations of the first X-variables. In the *score matrix* (**T**), with knowledge about the molecules, each molecule result is expressed by projections on to PCs instead of original variables: $\mathbf{X} = \mathbf{TP'} + \mathbf{E}$. Knowledge not enclosed in the matrices stays as *unexplained X-variance* in a *residual matrix* (**E**). Each PC_i results a novel coordinate stated as a linear combination of the first characteristics x_j: $PC_i = \Sigma_j b_{ij} x_j$. The novel coordinates PC_i result *scores* or *factors* whereas the coefficients b_{ij} result the *loadings*. The scores are sorted consistently with the knowledge regarding the entire variability between molecules. The *score-score plots* present the places of the molecules in the novel coordinate scheme, whereas the *loading-loading*

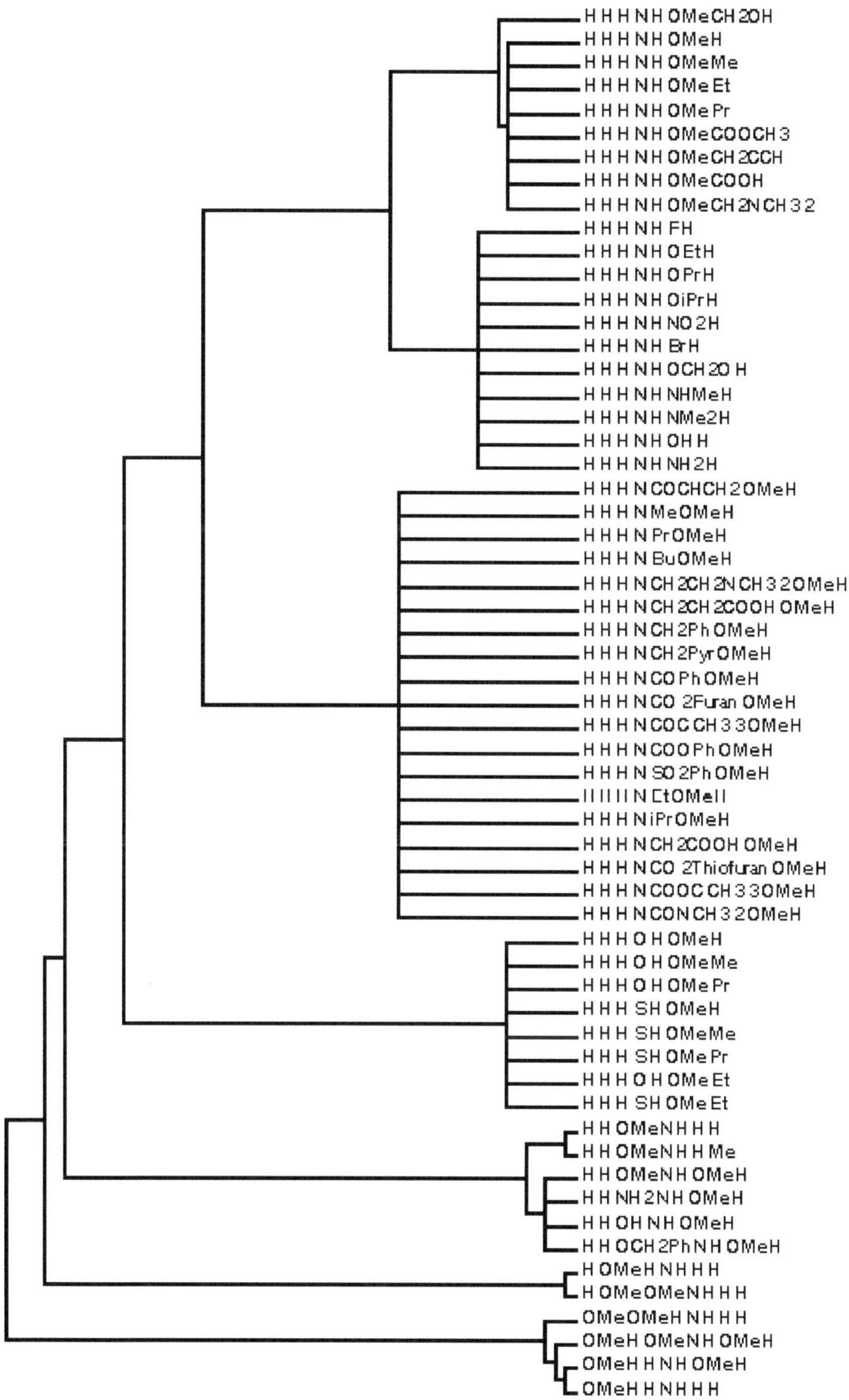

Figure 3. Dendrogram of TMP ring/indole ring/C=O bridge as MKN-45 inhibitors.

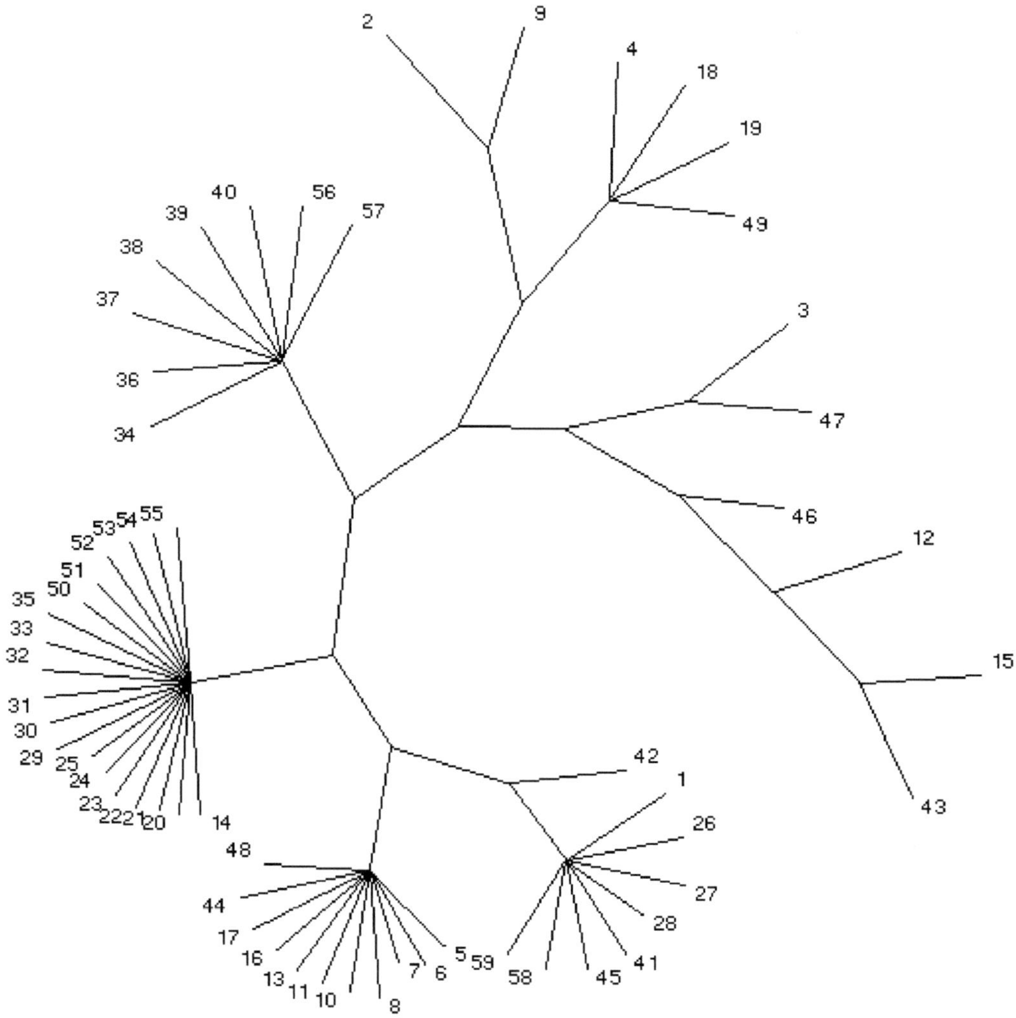

Figure 4. Radial tree of TMP ring/indole ring/C=O bridge as MKN-45 inhibitors.

plots display the position of the properties that correspond to the molecules in the novel coordinate scheme. The PCs show a pair of features. (1) The PCs result taken out in decreasing sequence of significance: the first PC encloses more knowledge than the second one, the second more than the third one, and so on. (2) Each PC results orthogonal to each other: no correlation exists between information contained in different PCs. A PCA was performed for TMPs. The importance of PCA factors F_{1-7} for $\{i_1,i_2,i_3,i_4,i_5,i_6,i_7\}$ was calculated. In particular, the use of the first factor F_1 explains 27% of the variability of data (73% error), the combined application of the first two factors $F_{1/2}$ accounts for 45% of variance (55% error), the utilization of the first three factors F_{1-3} justifies 60% of variability (40% error), etc. Factor loadings of PCA were computed. Profile of PCA F_1–F_2 for vector property was calculated. For F_1, variable i_6 shows the maximum weight in the profile; notwithstanding, F_1 is not able to be downgraded to two variables $\{i_5,i_6\}$ devoid of a 48% error. For F_2, variable i_4 presents the maximum weight and F_2

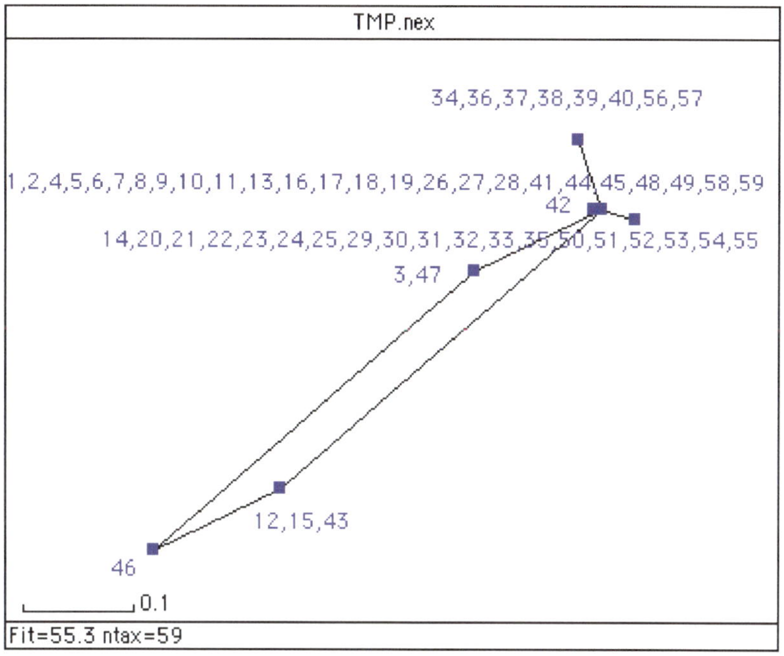

Figure 5. Splits graph of TMP ring/indole ring/C=O bridge as MKN-45 inhibitors.

is able to be downgraded to two variables $\{i_4,i_5\}$ with a 5% error. For F_3, variable i_7 assigns the maximum weight and F_3 is able to be downgraded to two variables $\{i_4,i_7\}$ with a 3% error. For F_4, variable i_3 consigns the maximum weight; however, F_4 is not able to be downgraded to two variables $\{i_2,i_3\}$ devoid of a 15% error. For F_5, variable i_1 represents the maximum weight and F_5 is able to be downgraded to two variables $\{i_1,i_6\}$ with a 6% error. For F_6, variable i_2 explains the maximum weight; notwithstanding, F_6 is not able to be downgraded to two variables $\{i_1,i_2\}$ devoid of a 25% error. For F_7, variable i_5 accounts for the maximum weight; nevertheless, F_7 is not able to be downgraded to two variables $\{i_5,i_6\}$ devoid of a 36% error. In PCA F_2–F_1 scores plot (**Figure 6**), TMPs with the same vector property collapse: (1,26–28,41,45,58,59), (2,9), (4,18,19,49) (5–8,10,11,13,16,17,44,48), (14,20–25,29–33,35,50–55) and (34,36–40,56,57). Seven TMP classes are clearly distinguished: class 1 with 9 compounds ($0 < F_1 < F_2$, *right*), class 2 with 11 substances ($F_1 < F_2 \approx 0$, *middle*), class 3 with 19 molecules ($F_1 >> F_2$, *bottom right*), class 4 with 8 organics ($0 < F_1 << F_2$, *top*), class 5 (6 units, $F_1 < F_2 \approx 0$, *middle*), class 6 (2 units, $F_1 << F_2 < 0$, *left*) and class 7 (4 units, $F_1 < F_2 < 0$, *bottom*). The classification is in agreement with partial correlation diagram, dendrograms, radial tree, and splits graph.

From PCA factor loadings of TMPs, F_2–F_1 loadings plot (**Figure 7**) depicts the seven properties. In addition, as a complement to the scores plot for the loadings, it is confirmed that TMPs in class 1, located in the right side, present a contribution of R_3 = OMe situated in the same side. The TMPs in class 3 in the bottom have more pronounced contribution of X = N in the same location. Two classes of properties are clearly distinguished in the loadings plot: class 1 $\{R_1,R_4,R_2,R_3\}$ ($F_1 > F_2 > 0$, *right*) and class 2 $\{X,R_5,R_6\}$ ($F_1 < F_2$, *left*).

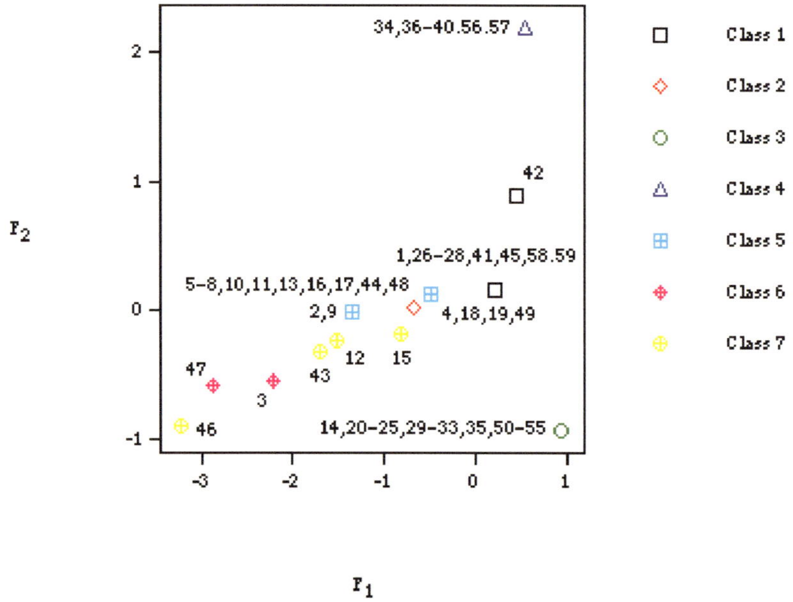

Figure 6. Principal component analysis F_2–F_1 scores plot for TMP ring/indole ring/C=O bridge.

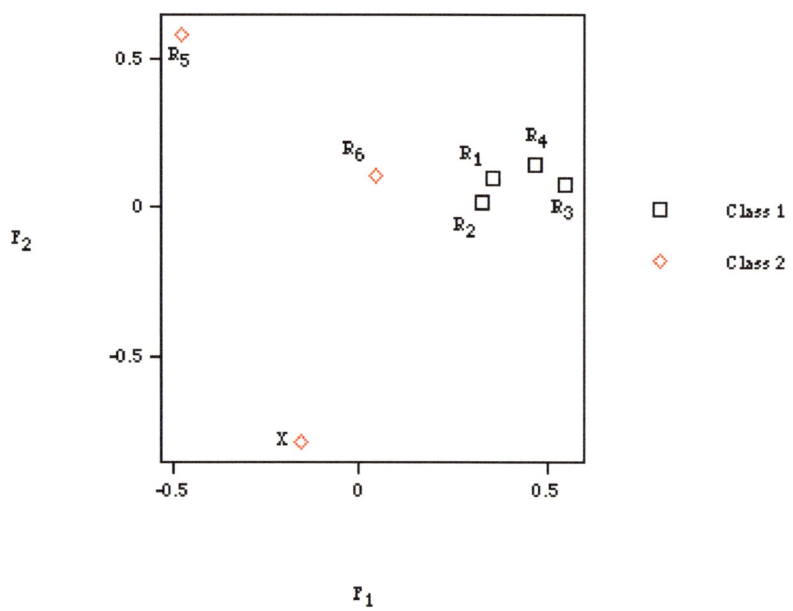

Figure 7. PCA F_2–F_1 loadings plot for TMP ring/indole ring/C=O bridge.

Instead of 59 TMPs in the $\mathfrak{R}^7$ space of seven vector properties, we consider seven properties in the $\mathfrak{R}^{59}$ space of 59 TMPs. The dendrogram for vector properties separates properties {R_1, R_4,R_2,R_3} (class 1) from {X,R_5,R_6} (class 2), in agreement with PCA loadings plot. The splits graph for properties indicates no conflicting relation between vector components, separating properties $\{R_1,R_4,R_2,R_3\}$ (class 1) from $\{X,R_5,R_6\}$ (class 2), in agreement with PCA loadings plot and dendrogram. A PCA was performed for the vector properties. The use of only the first factor F_1 explains 51% of variance (49% error), the combined application of the first two factors $F_{1/2}$ accounts for 71% of variability (29% error), the utilization of the first three factors F_{1-3} rationalizes 82% of variance (18% error), etc. In the PCA F_2–F_1 scores plot, property R_4 appears superimposed on R_1. Two groupings of properties are distinguished: class 1 $\{R_1,R_4,R_2,R_3\}$ ($F_1 > F_2$, *right*) and class 2 $\{X,R_5,R_6\}$ ($F_1 < F_2$, *left*), in agreement with PCA loadings plot, dendrogram and splits graph. Format for PT of TMPs (**Table 1**) indicates that TMPs are categorized first by i_1, then i_2, i_3, i_4, i_5, i_6, and i_7. Vertical groups result described by $\{i_1,i_2,i_3,i_4\}$ and horizontal periods, by $\{i_5,i_6,i_7\}$. Periods of eight elements are considered; e.g., group g0011 denotes $<i_1,i_2,i_3,i_4> = <0011>$: <0011100> ($R_1 \neq H$, $R_4 \neq H$, $R_2 = H$, $X = N$, $R_5 = H$, $R_3 \neq OMe$, $R_6 \neq CH_2$–OH), etc. The TMPs in the same column appear close in partial correlation diagram, dendrograms, radial tree, splits graph, and PCA scores.

The change of property P (inhibition of gastric cancer cell MKN-45) of vector $<i_1,i_2,i_3,i_4,i_5,i_6,i_7>$ is expressed in the decimal system $P = 10^6 i_1 + 10^5 i_2 + 10^4 i_3 + 10^3 i_4 + 10^2 i_5 + 10 i_6 + i_7$ *vs.* structural parameters $\{i_1,i_2,i_3,i_4,i_5,i_6,i_7\}$, for TMPs. The property was not used in the development of PT and serves to validate it. Most points appear superimposed, and lines $i_{2/6}$ on i_1 and i_7 on i_4. Results show the order of importance of parameters: $i_1 > i_2 > i_3 > i_4 > i_5 > i_6 > i_7$, in agreement with PT of properties with vertical groups defined by $\{i_1,i_2,i_3,i_4\}$ and horizontal periods by $\{i_5,i_6,i_7\}$. The variation property P of vector $<i_1,i_2,i_3,i_4,i_5,i_6,i_7>$ in base 10 *vs.* the number of group in PT, for TMPs, reveals minima corresponding to compounds with $<i_1,i_2,i_3,i_4>$ *ca.* <0011> (group g0011) and maxima *ca.* <1111> (group g1111). Periods p010, p100, p110, and p111 represent rows 1–4, respectively. For groups 3 and 6, period p110 is superimposed on p100, and for group 8, all periods coincide. The corresponding function $P(i_1,i_2,i_3,i_4,i_5,i_6,i_7)$ indicates a series of cyclic *waves* obviously controlled by minima or maxima, which propose a periodic performance that evokes the shape of a trigonometric function. For $<i_1,i_2,i_3,i_4,i_5,i_6,i_7>$, maximum results are obviously presented. The space in $<i_1,i_2,i_3,i_4,i_5,i_6,i_7>$ elements among every couple of successive maxima is eight, which agrees with TMP collections in consecutive periods. The maxima are in similar locations in the curve and are in phase. The typical points in phase have to match with the components in similar group in PT. For maxima $<i_1,i_2,i_3,i_4,i_5,i_6,i_7>$, there is consistency among the two descriptions; notwithstanding, the constancy is not universal. The assessment of the waves presents a pair of dissimilarities: (1) periods are incomplete and (2) periods 2 and 3 are somewhat staircase like. The most characteristic points of the plot are maxima that lie about group g1111. The values of $<i_1,i_2,i_3,i_4,i_5,i_6,i_7>$ are repeated as the periodic law (PL) states. An empirical function $P(p)$ reproduces different $<i_1,i_2,i_3,i_4,i_5,i_6,i_7>$ values; a minimum of $P(p)$ presents significance just if it is contrasted with the previous $P(p–1)$ and afterward $P(p + 1)$ points, necessitating to satisfy:

$$\begin{aligned} P_{\min}(p) &< P(p-1) \\ P_{\min}(p) &< P(p+1) \end{aligned} \tag{8}$$

Sequenced relationship (8) has to be done again at determined gaps peer to the dimension of the period and is equal to:

g0011	g0101	g0111	g1001
–OMe –OMe –H –N –H –H –H		–OMe –H –H –N –H –H –H	–H –OMe –OMe –N –H –H –H
	–OMe –H –OMe –N –H –OMe –H	–OMe –H –H –N –H –OMe –H	

g1011	g1101	g1110	g1111
			–H –H –H –N –CO–CH=CH_2 –OMe –H –H –H –H –N –Me –OMe –H –H –H –H –N –Pr –OMe –H –H –H –H –N –Bu –OMe –H –H –H –H –N –CH_2–CH_2–N$(CH_3)_2$ –OMe –H –H –H –H –N –CH_2–CH_2–CO–OH –OMe –H –H –H –H –N –CH_2–Ph –OMe –H –H –H –H –N –CH_2–Pyr –OMe –H –H –H –H –N –CO–Ph –OMe –H –H –H –H –N –CO–2-Furan –OMe –H –H –H –H –N –CO–C$(CH_3)_3$ –OMe –H –H –H –H –N –CO–O–Ph –OMe –H –H –H –H –N –SO_2–Ph –OMe –H –H –H –H –N –Et –OMe –H –H –H –H –N –*i*-Pr –OMe –H –H –H –H –N –CH_2–CO–OH –OMe –H –H –H –H –N –CO–2-Thiofuran –OMe –H –H –H –H –N –CO–O–C$(CH_3)_3$ –OMe –H –H –H –H –N –CO–N$(CH_3)_2$ –OMe –H
–H –OMe –H –N –H –H –H	–H –H –OMe –N –H –H –H –H –H –OMe –N –H –H –Me		–H –H –H –N –H –F –H –H –H –H –N –H –OEt –H –H –H –H –N –H –OPr –H –H –H –H –N –H –O-*i*-Pr –H –H –H –H –N –H –NO_2 –H –H –H –H –N –H –Br –H –H –H –H –N –H –O–CH_2–O– –H –H –H –H –N –H –NHMe –H –H –H –H –N –H –N$(Me)_2$ –H –H –H –H –N –H –OH –H –H –H –H –N –H –NH_2 –H
	–H –H –OMe –N –H –OMe –H –H –H –NH_2 –N –H –OMe –H –H –H –OH –N –H –OMe –H –H –H –O–CH_2–Ph –N –H –OMe –H	–H –H –H –O –H –OMe –H –H –H –H –O –H –OMe –Me –H –H –H –O –H –OMe –Pr	–H –H –H –N –H –OMe –H –H –H –H –N –H –OMe –Me –H –H –H –N –H –OMe –Et –H –H –H –N –H –OMe –Pr –H –H –H –N –H –OMe –CO–O–CH_3 –H –H –H –N –H –OMe

g1011	g1101	g1110	g1111
		–H –H –H –S –H –OMe –H –H –H –H –S –H –OMe –Me –H –H –H –S –H –OMe –Pr –H –H –H –O –H –OMe –Et –H –H –H –S –H –OMe –Et	$–CH_2–C≡CH$ –H –H –H –N –H –OMe –CO–OH –H –H –H –N –H –OMe $–CH_2–N(CH_3)_2$
			$–H –H –H –N –H –OMe –CH_2–OH$

Table 1. Periodic properties for 2-phenylindole-3-carbaldehyde derivatives.

$$\begin{aligned} P_{\min}(p) - P(p-1) < 0 \\ P(p+1) - P_{\min}(p) > 0 \end{aligned} \tag{9}$$

Because relationship (9) is just suitable for minima, additional universal others are wanted for all positions p; $D(p) = P(p + 1) - P(p)$ differences are computed by allocating each value to TMP p:

$$D(p) = P(p+1) - P(p) \tag{10}$$

In the place of $D(p)$, the values of $R(p) = P(p + 1)/P(p)$ are obtained by assigning $R(p)$ to TMP p; whether PL is universal, components in similar group in equivalent locations in dissimilar periodic waves assure:

either

$$D(p) > 0 \text{ or } D(p) < 0 \tag{11}$$

either

$$R(p) > 1 \text{ or } R(p) < 1 \tag{12}$$

Notwithstanding, the outcomes demonstrate that this is not the case, so PL is not universal but with anomalies. The change of $D(p)$ *vs.* group number shows that for group 6, periods p100 and p110 collapse. It introduces lack of consistency among $<i_1,i_2,i_3,i_4,i_5,i_6,i_7>$ Cartesian and PT charts. Whether constancy were exact, every position in each period present similar sign: in general, a tendency exists in the positions to provide $D(p) > 0$ for the lower groups but not for group 8; however, the latter results should be taken with care because $D(p)$ are calculated using data from the next period. In detail, irregularities exist in which TMPs for successive periods are not always in phase. The change of $R(p)$ *vs.* group number shows that for groups 3 and 6, periods p100 and p110 collapse, and, for group 8, all periods coincide, confirming the lack of steadiness among

Cartesian and PT representations. Whether control were precise or not, every position in every period presents $R(p)$ either smaller or larger than one. A tendency exists in the positions to provide $R(p) > 1$ for the lower groups but not for group 8; however, the latter should be taken with care because $R(p)$ are calculated from the next period. Confirmed incongruities exist in which TMPs for successive periods are not always in phase.

4. Conclusion

1. Several criteria were selected to reduce analysis to manage quantity of trimethoxyphenyl, indole, carbonyl bridge antitubulins referred to structural parameters related to positions $R_{1–4}$ on benzo, $R_{5/6}$ on pyridine, and heteroatom X in indole. Molecular *structural elements* were *ranked* according to inhibitory activity: $R_1 > R_4 > R_2 > X > R_5 > R_3 > R_6$. In compound 42, $R_1 = R_4 = R_2 = R_5 =$ H, X = N, $R_3 =$ OMe and $R_6 = CH_3–OH$ <1,111,111>, which was selected as *reference*. Many classification algorithms are based on *information entropy*. For moderate-sized sets, an excessive number of results appear compatible with data and suffer a combinatorial explosion; however, after the *equipartition conjecture,* one has a selection criterion, according to which the best configuration is that in which entropy production is most uniformly distributed. Method avoids the problem of continuum variables because for compound with constant <1,111,111> vector, null standard deviation causes Pearson correlation coefficient of one. Classification is in agreement with the analyses by principal components.

2. Code MolClas is an easy, dependable, effective, and quick process for the classification of molecules founded on the conjecture of the equipartition of the production of the entropy of information. The code was developed not just to examine the conjecture of equipartition but, in addition, to discover the world of the classification of molecules.

3. The periodic law does not convince the category of the laws of physics: (1) antitubulin inhibitory powers do not result done again; maybe their chemical nature; (2) sequence relations are done again with exemptions. The examination compels the declaration: relationships that whichever molecule p presents with its neighbor $p + 1$ are more or less done again for each period. Periodicity result is not universal; notwithstanding, if a usual order of molecules are agreed, the rule should be phenomenological. The antiproliferative potency did not generate the table of periodic classification and serves to confirm it. The examination of other antitubulin features would give an insight into the achievable generalization of the periodic table.

Acknowledgements

The authors thank support from Generalitat Valenciana (Project No. PROMETEO/2016/094) and Valencia Catholic University *Saint Vincent Martyr* (Project No. PRUCV/2015/617).

Author details

Francisco Torrens[1]* and Gloria Castellano[2]

*Address all correspondence to: torrens@uv.es

1 Institute for Molecular Science, University of Valencia, Valencia, Spain

2 Department of Experimental Sciences and Mathematics, Faculty of Veterinary and Experimental Sciences, Valencia Catholic University Saint Vincent Martyr, Valencia, Spain

References

[1] DeMartino G, Edler MC, LaRegina G, Coluccia A, Barbera MC, Barrow D, Nicholson RI, Chiosis G, Brancale A, Hamel E, Artico M, Silvestri R. New arylthioindoles: Potent inhibitors of tubulin polymerization. 2. Structure-activity relationships and molecular modeling studies. Journal of Medicinal Chemistry. 2006;**49**:947-954

[2] DeMartino G, LaRegina G, Coluccia A, Edler MC, Barbera MC, Brancale A, Wilcox E, Hamel E, Artico M, Silvestri R. Arylthioindoles, potent inhibitors of tubulin polymerization. Journal of Medicinal Chemistry. 2004;**47**:6120-6123

[3] Chang JY, Hsieh HP, Chang CY, Hsu KS, Chiang YF, Chen CM, Kuo CC, Liou JP. 7-Aroyl-aminoindoline-1-sulfonamides as a novel class of potent antitubulin agents. Journal of Medicinal Chemistry. 2006;**49**:6656-6659

[4] Liou JP, Chang YL, Kuo FM, Chang CW, Tseng HY, Wang CC, Yang YN, Chang JY, Lee SJ, Hsieh HP. Concise synthesis and structure-activity relationships of combretastatin A-4 analogues, 1-aroylindoles and 3-aroylindoles, as novel classes of potent antitubulin agents. Journal of Medicinal Chemistry. 2004;**47**:4247-4257

[5] Chang JY, Yang MF, Chang CY, Chen CM, Kuo CC, Liou JP. 2-amino and 2′-aminocombretastatin derivatives as potent antimitotic agents. Journal of Medicinal Chemistry. 2006; **49**:6412-6415

[6] Liou JP, Mahindroo N, Chang CW, Guo FM, Lee SWH, Tan UK, Yeh TK, Kuo CC, Chang YW, Lu PH, Tung YS, Lin KT, Chang JY, Hsieh HP. Structure–activity relationship studies of 3-aroylindoles as potent antimitotic agents. ChemMedChem. 2006;**1**:1106-1118

[7] Rappl C, Barbier P, Bourgarel-Rey V, Gregoire C, Gilli R, Carre M, Combes S, Finet JP, Peyrot V. Interaction of 4-arylcoumarin analogues of combretastatins with microtubule network of HBL100 cells and binding to tubulin. Biochemistry. 2006;**45**:9210-9218

[8] Romagnoli R, Baraldi PG, Remusat V, Carrion MD, Cara CL, Petri D, Fruttarolo F, Pavani MG, Tabrizi MA, Tolomeo M, Grimaudo S, Balzarini J, Jordan MA, Hamel E. Synthesis and biological evaluation of 2-(3′,4′,5′-trimethoxybenzoyl)-3-amino 5-aryl thiophenes as a new class of tubulin inhibitors. Journal of Medicinal Chemistry. 2006;**49**:6425-6428

[9] Nguyen TL, McGrath C, Hermone AR, Burnett JC, Zaharevitz DW, Day BW, Wipf P, Hamel E, Gussio R. A common pharmacophore for a diverse set of colchicine site inhibitors using a structure-based approach. Journal of Medicinal Chemistry. 2005;**48**:6107-6116

[10] Kim DY, Kim KH, Kim ND, Lee KY, Han CK, Yoon JH, Moon SK, Lee SS, Seong BL. Design and biological evaluation of novel tubulin inhibitors as antimitotic agents using a pharmacophore binding model with tubulin. Journal of Medicinal Chemistry. 2006;**49**: 5664-5670

[11] Liou JP, Wu ZY, Kuo CC, Chang CY, Lu PY, Chen CM, Hsieh HP, Chang JY. Discovery of 4-amino and 4-hydroxy-1-aroylindoles as potent tubulin polymerization inhibitors. Journal of Medicinal Chemistry. 2008;**51**:4351-4355

[12] Hsieh HP, Liou JP, Mahindroo N. Pharmaceutical design of antimitotic agents based on combretastatins. Current Pharmaceutical Design. 2005;**11**:1655-1677

[13] Mahindroo N, Liou JP, Chang JY, Hsieh HP. Antitubulin agents for the treatment of cancer – A medicinal chemistry update. Expert Opinion on Therapeutic Patents. 2006;**16**:647-691

[14] Ducki S, Mackenzie G, Lawrence NJ, Snyder JP. Quantitative structure-activity relationship (5D-QSAR) study of combretastatin-like analogues as inhibitors of tubulin assembly. Journal of Medicinal Chemistry. 2005;**48**:457-465

[15] Bellina F, Cauteruccio S, Monti S, Rossi R. Novel imidazole-based combretastatin A-4 analogues: Evaluation of their in vitro antitumor activity and molecular modeling study of their binding to the colchicine site of tubulin. Bioorganic & Medicinal Chemistry Letters. 2006;**16**:5757-5762

[16] Brown ML, Rieger JM, Macdonald TL. Comparative molecular field analysis of colchicine inhibition and tubulin polymerization for combretastatins binding to the colchicine binding site on beta-tubulin. Bioorganic & Medicinal Chemistry. 2000;**8**:1433-1441

[17] Pan X, Tan N, Zeng G, Han H, Huang H. 3D-QSAR and docking studies of aldehyde inhibitors of human cathepsin K. Bioorganic & Medicinal Chemistry. 2006;**14**:2771-2778

[18] Wolohan P, Reichert DE. CoMFA and docking study of novel estrogen receptor subtype selective ligands. Journal of Computer-Aided Molecular Design. 2003;**17**:313-328

[19] Liu H, Huang X, Shen J, Luo X, Li M, Xiong B, Chen G, Shen J, Yang Y, Jiang H, Chen K. Inhibitory mode of 1,5-diarylpyrazole derivatives against cyclooxygenase-2 and cyclooxygenase-1: Molecular docking and 3D QSAR analyses. Journal of Medicinal Chemistry. 2002;**45**:4816-4827

[20] Cheng F, Shen J, Luo X, Zhu W, Gu J, Ji R, Jiang H, Chen K. Molecular docking and 3-D-QSAR studies on the possible antimalarial mechanism of artemisinin analogues. Bioorganic & Medicinal Chemistry. 2002;**10**:2883-2891

[21] Du J, Qin J, Liu H, Yao X. 3D-QSAR and molecular docking studies of selective agonists for the thyroid hormone receptor beta. Journal of Molecular Graphics and Modelling. 2008;**27**:95-104

[22] Lin IH, Hsu CC, Wang SH, Hsieh HP, Sun YC. Comparative molecular field analysis of anti-tubulin agents with indole ring binding at the colchicine binding site. Journal of Theoretical and Computational Chemistry. 2010;**9**:279-291

[23] Cramer RD, III, Patterson DE, Bunce JD. Comparative molecular field analysis (CoMFA). 1. Effect of shape on binding of steroids to carrier proteins. Journal of the American Chemical Society 1988;**110**:5959-5967

[24] Halder AK, Adhikari N, Jha T. Comparative QSAR modelling of 2-phenylindole-3-carbaldehyde derivatives as potential antimitotic agents. Bioorganic & Medicinal Chemistry Letters. 2009;**19**:1737-1739

[25] Gajiwaja KS, Wu JC, Christensen J, Deshmukh GD, Diehl W, DiNitto JP, English JM, Greig MJ, He YA, Jacques SL, Lunney EA, McTigue M, Molina D, Quenzer T, Wells PA, Yu X, Zhang Y, Zou A, Emmett MR, Marshall AG, Zhang HM, Demetri GD. KIT kinase mutants show unique mechanisms of drug resistance to imatinib and sunitinib in gastrointestinal stromal tumor patients. Proceedings of the National Academy of Sciences of the United States of America. 2009;**106**:1542-1547

[26] Marimuthu A, Jacob HKC, Jakharia A, Subbannayya Y, Keerthikumar S, Kashyap MK, Goel R, Balakrishnan L, Dwivedi S, Pathare S, Dikshit JB, Maharudraiah J, Singh S, Kumar GSS, Vijayakumar M, Kumar KVV, Premalatha CS, Tata P, Hariharan R, Roa JC, Prasad TSK, Chaerkady R, Kumar RV, Pandey A. Gene expression profiling of gastric cancer. Journal of Proteomics and Bioinformatics. 2011;**4**(4):74-82

[27] Santavy F. Substanzen der herbstzeitlose und ihre derivate. XXII. Photochemische produkte des colchicins und einige seiner derivate. Collection of Czechoslovak Chemical Communications. 1951;**16**:665-675

[28] Andreu JM, Perez-Ramirez B, Gorbunoff MJ, Ayala D, Timasheff SN. Role of the colchicine ring a and its methoxy groups in the binding to tubulin and microtubule inhibition. Biochemistry. 1998;**37**:8356-8368

[29] Nunez J, Fellous A, Francon J, Lennon AM. Competitive inhibition of colchicine binding to tubulin by microtubule-associated proteins. Proceedings of the National Academy of Sciences of the United States of America. 1979;**76**:86-90

[30] Lee RM, Gewirtz DA. Colchicine site inhibitors of microtubule integrity as vascular disrupting agents. Drug Development Research. 2008;**69**:352-358

[31] Bhattacharyya B, Panda D, Gupta S, Banerjee M. Anti-mitotic activity of colchicine and the structural basis for its interaction with tubulin. Medicinal Research Reviews. 2008;**28**: 155-183

[32] Jordan MA, Wilson L. Microtubules as a target for anticancer drugs. Nature Reviews. Cancer. 2004;**4**:253-265

[33] Brancale A, Silvestri R. Indole, a core nucleus for potent inhibitors of tubulin polymerization. Medicinal Research Reviews. 2007;**27**:209-238

[34] Sengupta S, Thomas SA. Drug target interaction of tubulin-binding drugs in cancer therapy. Expert Review of Anticancer Therapy. 2006;**6**:1433-1447

[35] Varmuza K. Pattern Recognition in Chemistry. New York: Springer; 1980

[36] Benzecri JP. L'Analyse des Données. Paris: Dunod; 1984. Vol. 1

[37] Tondeur D, Kvaalen E. Equipartition of entropy production. An optimality criterion for transfer and separation processes. Industrial & Engineering Chemistry Fundamentals. 1987;**26**:50-56

[38] Torrens F, Periodic CG. Classification of local anaesthetics (procaine analogues). International Journal of Molecular Sciences. 2006;**7**:12-34

[39] Castellano-Estornell G, Torrens-Zaragozá F. Local anaesthetics classified using chemical structural indicators. Nereis. 2009;**2009**(2):7-17

[40] Torrens F, Castellano G. Using chemical structural indicators for periodic classification of local anaesthetics. Int. J. Chemoinf. Chemical Engineer. 2011;**1**(2):15-35

[41] Torrens F, Castellano G. Table of periodic properties of human immunodeficiency virus inhibitors. International Journal of Computational Intelligence in Bioinformatics and Systems Biology. 2010;**1**:246-273

[42] Torrens F, Molecular CG. Classification of thiocarbamates with cytoprotection activity against human immunodeficiency virus. International Journal of Chemical Modeling. 2011;**3**:269-296

[43] Torrens F, Molecular CG. Classification of styrylquinolines as human immunodeficiency virus integrase inhibitors. International Journal of Chemical Modeling. 2014;**6**:347-376

[44] Torrens F, Castellano G. Modelling of complex multicellular systems: Tumour–immune cells competition. Chemistry Central Journal. 2009;**3**(Suppl. I):75–1-1

[45] Torrens F, Castellano G. Information theoretic entropy for molecular classification: Oxadiazolamines as potential therapeutic agents. Current Computer-Aided Drug Design. 2013;**9**:241-253

[46] Kaufmann A. Introduction à la Théorie des Sous-ensembles Flous. Paris: Masson; 1975. Vol. 3

[47] Cox E. The Fuzzy Systems Handbook. New York: Academic; 1994

[48] Kundu S. The min–max composition rule and its superiority over the usual max–min composition rule. Fuzzy Sets and Systems. 1998;**93**:319-329

[49] G. Lambert-Torres G, Pereira Pinto JO, Borges da Silva LE. In: Wiley Encyclopedia of Electrical and Electronics Engineering. New York: Wiley; 1999

[50] Shannon CE. A mathematical theory of communication: Part I, discrete noiseless systems. Bell System Technical Journal. 1948;**27**:379-423

[51] Shannon CE. A mathematical theory of communication. Part II, The discrete channel with noise. Bell System Technical Journal. 1948;**27**:623-656

[52] Neural WH. Network learning and statistics. AI Expert. 1989;**4**(12):48-52

[53] Kullback S. Information Theory and Statistics. New York: Wiley; 1959

[54] Iordache O, Corriou JP, Garrido-Sánchez L, Fonteix C, Tondeur D. Neural network frames. Application to biochemical kinetic diagnosis. Computers and Chemical Engineering. 1993; **17**:1101-1113

[55] Wildenhain J, FitzGerald N, Tyers M. MolClass: A web portal to interrogate diverse small molecule screen datasets with different computational models. Bioinformatics. 2012;**28**: 2200-2201

[56] Tryon RCA. Multivariate analysis of the risk of coronary heart disease in Framingham. Journal of Chronic Diseases. 1939;**20**:511-524

[57] Jarvis RA, Patrick EA. Clustering using a similarity measure based on shared nearest neighbors. IEEE Transactions on Computers. 1973;**C22**:1025-1034

[58] Eisen MB, Spellman PT, Brown PO, Botstein D. Cluster analysis and display of genome-wide expression patterns. Proceedings of the National Academy of Sciences of the United States of America. 1998;**95**:14863-14868

[59] Page RDM. Program TreeView. Glasgow: Universiy of Glasgow; 2000

[60] Huson DH. SplitsTree: Analyzing and visualizing evolutionary data. Bioinformatics. 1998;**14**:68-73

[61] Hotelling H. Analysis of a complex of statistical variables into principal components. Journal of Education & Psychology. 1933;**24**:417-441

[62] Kramer R. Chemometric Techniques for Quantitative Analysis. New York: Marcel Dekker; 1998

[63] Patra SK, Mandal AK, Pal MK. State of aggregation of bilirubin in aqueous solution: Principal component analysis approach. Journal of Photochemistry and Photobiology A. 1999;**122**:23-31

[64] Jolliffe IT. Principal Component Analysis. New York: Springer; 2002

[65] Xu J, Hagler A. Chemoinformatics and drug discovery. Molecules. 2002;**7**:566-600

[66] Shaw PJA. Multivariate Statistics for the Environmental Sciences. New York:Hodder-Arnold; 2003

Chapter 5

Multifunctional Polymeric Enveloped Nanocarriers: Targeting Extracellular and Intracellular Barriers

Maria Hassan Kiani, Masoom Yasinzai and Gul Shahnaz

Additional information is available at the end of the chapter

http://dx.doi.org/10.5772/intechopen.74624

Abstract

Over the past several years, employment of multifunctional polymeric excipients-based nanoparticles for controlled and targeted drug delivery of therapeutic modalities to mucosal membrane-based organelles and systemic circulation has gained enormous interest. Because they promise to resolve numerous key therapeutical issues associated with current clinical practice including low treatment efficacy and significant side effects. Potential controlled and targeted drug delivery systems, therefore, should be able to overcome not only extracellular barriers but also intracellular barriers. Extracellularly, targeted nanocarriers ought to provide extended circulation time, selective binding to the targeted mucosal tissues, long residence time at the site of absorption, and controlled drug release. Intracellularly, the targeted nanocarriers should offer cellular uptake, cellular localization, and endosomal release. Hence, this chapter will provide an overview of the unique chemistry of multifunctional polymeric enveloped diverse nanocarriers such as dendrimers, semiconducting polymer dots, quantum dots, carbon dots, and magnetic as versatile platform addressing both extracellular and intracellular barriers.

Keywords: polymeric nanocarriers, extracellular drug targeting, intracellular drug targeting, carbon dots, polymer dots, quantum dots, magnetic nanoparticles

1. Introduction

Targeted drug delivery has been massively investigated because of their potential to overcome hurdles of conventional therapy [1]. Administration of drug selectively at desired site ensures the maximum amount of drug to be available at that locality. Moreover, lesser absorption of drug systemically minimizes the potential for unwanted effects. To target a drug so that it may avoid its uptake by off target tissues or cell and allow its residence at desired site for longer period of time, it is usually escorted with some targeting agent. These targeting molecules can be receptor-specific ligands, vehicles, or biological molecules [2].

Nanocarriers have revolutionized therapeutic approaches by providing numerous means for drug targeting. Nanocarriers have employed various approaches to target drug to a specific organ, tissue, cell, or organelle. The therapeutic efficacy of these carrier systems is highly dependent on their entry into target sites. It has been studied that passage of particles across endothelial cells requires their size to be less than 100 nm approximately [3]. This limits the greater-sized particles to extravagate into tissues having compromised endothelial arrangement. Nanostructures with hydrophobic outer surface have been observed to undergo phagocytosis after being opsonized [4].

Various polymers with diverse chemical nature and various activities and characteristics have been explored to design nanocarriers for delivery of drug molecules. Among them, biodegradable polymers have been of particular interest. Both natural and synthetic biodegradable polymers have been exploited to functionalize nanoparticles exploiting diverse approaches to deliver drug in an effective manner to its target site [1]. Such functionalized polymeric nanostructures (also known as multiplex nanoparticles) have been widely investigated as an effective carrier for a wide variety of drugs as well as biological molecules such as DNA and proteins [1]. Current research has been precisely focused on the use of biodegradable polymers that have shown great promise in modifying the delivery of drug as well as tissue engineering. Such polymers have shown to provide extended and targeted drug release for days to weeks as well as shown great promise for intracellular transport of drugs [5].

Various treatment modalities require intracellular delivery of drug as the causative agent is harboring within cell. This is the case commonly associated with infectious diseases such as tuberculosis, leishmaniasis, and leprosy, where the pathogen invades macrophages. Therefore, complete eradication requires utmost delivery of drug at right concentration to infected cells. Certain other conditions also require delivery of therapeutic agents into cytoplasm where they can target various cellular organelles such as endoplasmic reticulum, mitochondria, nucleus, and lysosomes [6]. This has found particular interest in gene therapy for targeting cellular genome [7] as well as drug targeting for the treatment of cancer and lysosomal storage disease [6]. Intracellular transport has also been widely appreciated for bioimaging and biosensing both *in vitro* and *in vivo*.

2. Intracellular drug targeting

Entry or transport of drug into the cell has never been easy and thus widely explored [6]. Cells offer several mechanisms to allow ingress of drug carriers prominently comprising endocytosis. Internalization of drug into cells may either obey receptor-dependent endocytosis or receptor-independent pathway as shown in **Figure 1**. Combining small drug molecules with macromolecular carriers restricts their entry into highly perfused tissues, thus averting

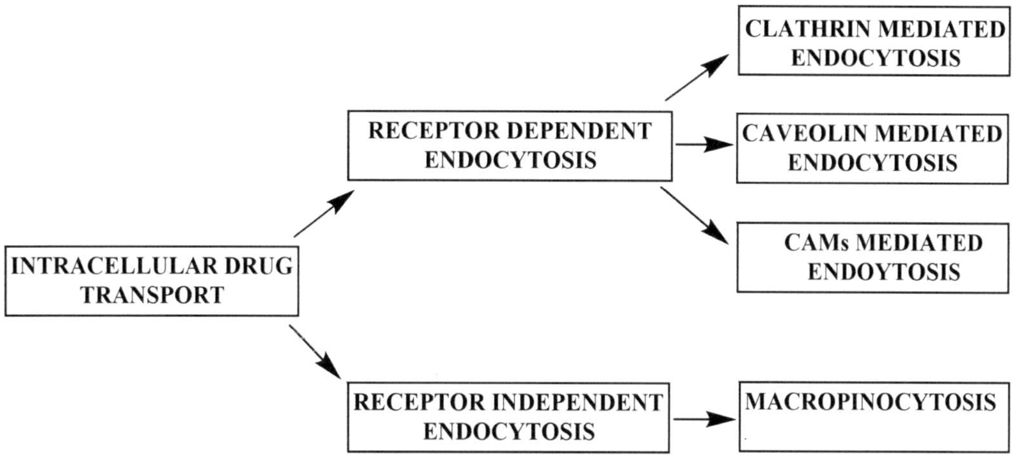

Figure 1. Pathways adopted for intracellular drug transport.

untoward side effects [2]. Macromolecules (proteins, peptides, DNA, etc.) are not allowed by lipophilic biological membranes to enter into cytoplasm. Such molecules may follow active transport involving endocytosis via cell surface receptors [6]. This receptor-mediated endocytosis offers a faster course for drug internalization in contrast to untargeted conjugates. These receptors have been located on surface of cells as well as accompany intracellular membranes [8].

2.1. Clathrin-associated, receptor-mediated endocytosis

The bases on which molecules are sorted to follow either clathrin-dependent or clathrin-independent pay are still not fully understood. However, it has been found that some specialized lipid domains are involved in membrane organization, sorting, and signal transduction in clathrin-independent endocytosis [9]. Ligand-associated drug carriers may bind to specific cell receptors that get assembled into particular areas of plasma membrane termed as coated pits. These regions (diameter 0.1 μm approx.) have been explained as plasma membrane invaginations with fuzzy cytoplasmic coat. This coat is mainly composed of clathrin protein present at cytoplasmic periphery of membrane and serves as major route for cellular internalization [10] as depicted in **Figure 2**. These coated pits allow intracellular vesicle formation in less than 1 min of time that is much faster than other mechanisms of endocytosis. A protein known as adaptin is responsible for polymerization of clathrin in the form of polyhedral lattice scaffold by binding with cell surface receptors. Two other proteins amphiphysin and endophilin get neighboring membrane into close vicinity. Dynamin (a cytosolic GTPase) gathers around the neckline of budding vesicle followed by its scission and intracellular discharge [2]. After intracellular entry of vesicle, an uncoating protein (heat shock protein; hsc70) causes the clathrin coat to shed of. At this stage, endocytosis trafficking of endosomal content decides the fate of therapeutic agent delivered. Endosomes may end up into lysosomes that may lead to degradation of drug or may be safely released into cytoplasm to reach desired organelle [6].

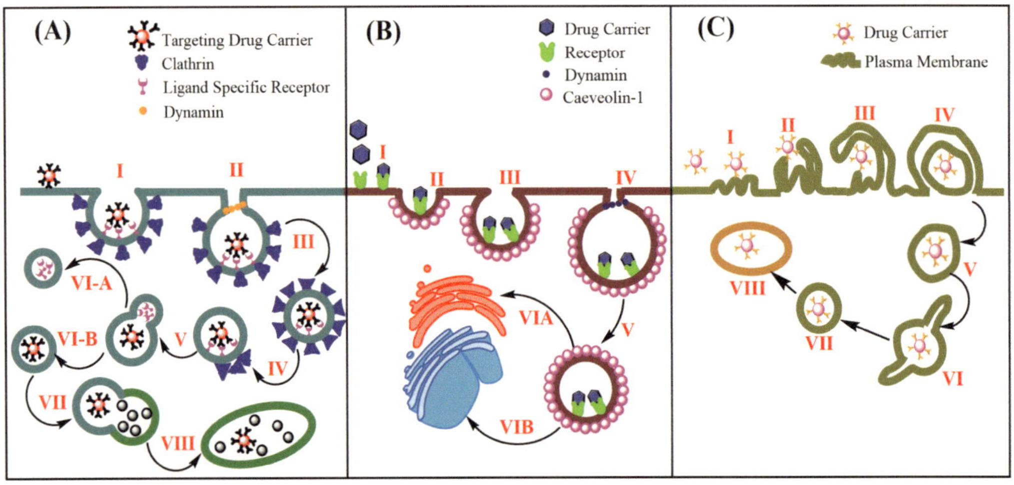

Figure 2. (A) Clathrin-dependent receptor-mediated endocytosis, I—entry of targeting drug carrier in clathrin-coated pits and binding with ligand-specific receptor; II—dynamin-associated endocytosis; III—formation of clathrin-coated vesicle; IV—shedding of clathrin coat; V—early endosomal sorting and uncoupling of ligand-receptor; VI-A—formation of late endosome; VI-B—formation of transport vesicle; VII—fusion of lysosome with transport vesicle; VIII—formation of endolysosome. (B) Caveolin-dependent, receptor-mediated endocytosis, I—interaction of ligand with receptor; II—movement of receptor ligand complex toward caveolar invagination; III—retention of receptor ligand complex in caveolar invagination; IV—dynamin-associated caveolar endocytosis; V—formation of caveosome; VI-A and VI-B—transport of drug carrier to endoplasmic reticulum or Golgi apparatus, respectively. (C) Macropinocytosis, I—movement of drug carrier toward membrane ruffling; II—rearrangement of cytoskeleton, folding of ruffle around drug carrier; IV—internalization; V—formation of macropinosome; VI—early maturation of macropinosome; VII—late endosome; VIII—endolysosome.

2.2. Cell adhesion molecule (CAM)-mediated endocytosis

Drug targeting has also been investigated using cell adhesion molecules (CAMs). Recently, integrins and cadherins have been found to internalize their ligand into intracellular milieu. Thus, many cell adhesion peptides such as arginylglycylaspartic acid (RGD) [11] and peptides derived from intercellular adhesion molecule 1 (ICAM-1) and lymphocyte function-associated antigen 1 (LFA-1) sequences that bind to specific integrins have been extensively investigated for targeting tumor and vascular endothelial cells and suppressed progression of autoimmune disorders [12]. CAMs undergo cellular internalization while they are recycled via clathrin-coated pits and thus can be useful in cell-specific drug targeting through specific peptides. Such peptides are usually derived from proteins comprising extracellular matrix, immunoglobulins superfamily, and integrins. Integrins have also been associated with cellular uptake of certain viruses and bacteria through surface interactions at unique regions and initiate transduction pathways [13].

2.3. Caveolin-dependent, receptor-mediated endocytosis

Another version for cellular internalization of drug carriers is caveolin-mediated endocytosis. This process is sensitive to temperature and also dependent on ATP and sulphydral reagents [14]. Caveolin-1 is a protein associated with flask-shaped invaginations making up greater than 10% of endothelial cell membrane. Only cells expressing caveolin-1 protein develop caveolar invaginations [15]. Ligand after association with plasma membrane moves along it toward caveolar invagination, where being retained for some time internalization occurs via certain unidentified receptor as shown in **Figure 2**. The presence of GTPase dynamin has suggested involvement of caveolae in membrane internalization [9].

Folic acid, cholesterol, albumin complexes, and serum lipoproteins are commonly encountered ligands internalized via caveolae-dependent endocytosis. These ligands have been considered as attractive candidates for drug targeting especially to intracellular organelles. Caveolar vesicles after getting internalized fuse with caveosomes following delivery of content at subcellular level bypassing acidic and degradative milieu of lysosomes [15]. Another mechanism suggested for caveolae-dependent internalization is 'potocytosis' that implies diffusion of smaller moieties into cytoplasm after interacting caveolae without membrane internalization [16]. One other associated pathway for cells without caveolae expression is 'lipid rafts'. These flat structures are composed of lipid- and protein-based assemblies that allow receptor-specific ligands to anchor on raft domain [15].

2.4. Macropinocytosis

Macropinocytosis employs distinct mechanism to transport molecules inside the cell without any direct coordination with receptors [17]. Macropinocytosis begins with actin polymerization at surface of cell membrane that is regulated by tyrosine kinase, epidermal growth factor, and platelet-derived growth factor receptors. This leads to increased ruffling at membrane surface and subsequent formation of macropinosomes (**Figure 2**). It involves absorption of molecules present in extracellular fluid (ECF) and seems to be a slower process as compared to RME. This process has sometimes shown to accompany receptor-mediated endocytosis; thus, absorption of receptor bound ligand and molecules in ECF may occur through clathrin-coated vesicles side by side. After entry of fluid vesicles, they are supposed to follow usual endolysosomal trafficking pathway [18]. Negative charge on membrane surface naturally favors positively charged molecules to reside there and eventually get internalized through fluid phase endocytosis. This phenomenon has been exploited by researches for intracellular delivery of drugs [19].

3. Extracellular drug targeting

Many targeting approaches utilize such mechanisms that exploit extracellular barriers to ensure efficient delivery of drugs. Nanocarriers following intravenous administration are rapidly recognized by reticuloendothelial system (liver and spleen macrophages), making it difficult for drug to reach its site of action at the minimum effective concentration [20]. This owes to opsonization of particle surface with certain plasma proteins (albumin, apolipoprotein-E, etc.) that make them recognizable by body's immune system and thus are rapidly evacuated from circulation. Therefore, the extent of opsonization will determine the fate of nanoparticles *in vivo* [21].

Recognition of nanoparticles by RES and their uptake by macrophages can be avoided by modifying surface properties of these carrier systems. One of such modifications is by making surface of nanoparticles to be very hydrophilic. This avoids adsorption of opsonins and ensures nanoparticles to pass unrecognized by RES [22]. Surface of nanoparticles has been made more hydrophilic by increasing the thickness of coating layer of poloxamer and poloxamine. Coating layers up to 10 nm were considered necessary to bypass RES [23].

Many drug molecules have shown poor penetration across the blood-brain barrier due to their inherent nature. These molecules have been successfully delivered to the brain when incorporated into nanocarriers [24]. Coated nanoparticles have been studied for delivery of drug into the brain. Polybutylcyanoacrylate (PBCA) nanoparticles coated with polysorbate-80 have been studied to improve penetration of drug across the blood-brain barrier [25]. In a study, transport of nanoparticles across BBB was investigated. Penetration of nanoparticles across BBB was three to four times increased when charged nanoparticles were coated with dipalmitoyl phosphatidyl choline and cholesterol-based lipid bilayer [26]. Multifunctional nanoparticles have also been investigated for delivery of proteins and peptides. These biological molecules are associated with rapid degradation at acidic pH of GIT and by activity of proteolytic enzymes that owe to their shorter half-life. Moreover, lesser partition coefficient and diffusivity make their movement difficult across biological membranes. These limitations can be conquered using functionalized polymeric nanoparticulate drug delivery systems [27]. Properties of PLGA matrices have been modified through hydrogel systems to deliver proteins and peptides. Bovine serum albumin was loaded in poly vinyl alcohol nanoparticles, which were then incorporated into PLGA microspheres and characterized to release the protein for more than 2 months [28]. Poly(isobutyl cyanoacrylate) nanocapsules have also been investigated for oral delivery of insulin [29].

Sustained release of drugs has also been achieved using various functionalized nanocarriers. Poly DL-lactic acid (PLA) nanoparticles have been used to provide sustained release of savoxepine following intramuscular and intravenous administrations [30]. Damge and his coworkers have successfully developed nanocapsules for sustained delivery of insulin. About 100 U/kg of insulin-loaded nanocapsules were effective to reduce blood glucose level for 6 days by 25% on oral administration to diabetic rats [31]. Colloidal suspension of docetaxel-loaded nanospheres has been prepared using PLA and PLGA to study sustained release of drug after intravenous administration [32]. PEG-grafted polyamidoamine (PAMAM) dendrimers were used to control the release of adriamycin and methotrexate [33]. Mu and Feng have used d-α-tocopheryl polyethylene glycol 1000 succinate (TPGS) to prepare controlled release paclitaxel nanoparticles with high encapsulation efficiency [34].

4. Nanocarriers for intracellular and extracellular targeting

Scientists have extensively explored a wide range of drug carriers at nanoscale extending from highly simple to complex geometries. Other than polymeric nanostructures, several lipids-based structures have been investigated for drug delivery, among which liposomes hold a noticeable status. Owing to their resemblance to lipid bilayer structure, they have been studied for a wide range of therapeutic applications (antivirals, antimicrobials, antitubercular drugs, biological molecules, and gene therapeutics) by offering enhanced accumulation and reduced toxicity at targeted site. However, reduced stability and trouble in immobilization of vector molecules on exterior of liposomes have led to exploration of other more useful nanocarriers [35]. Nanodots have exhibited great promise in therapeutics owing to diverse physicochemical properties, functionalization opportunities, and contenting stability attributes, which make them excellent candidate for bioimaging along with drug delivery. They have also been found substantially successful in photodynamic therapy in treatment of tumors [36]. Further, our discussion will be focused on multifunctional polymeric nanocarriers including dendrimers, various nanodot structures, and magnetic nanoparticles with reference to their application in intracellular and extracellular targeting for diagnostics and therapeutics.

4.1. Dendrimers

Dendrimers are three-dimensional, globular structures consisting of highly branched, repeating, and controllable peripheral functionalities originating from a central core [37]. These structures are assembled in layered fashion from core by repetition of two sequential reaction steps. Origination of a new branching point in layer leads to creation of a new generation (denoted as G). Thus, a regular dendrimer structure is usually composed of three major elements, i.e., a central core, branched units, and surface groups [38]. Such a diverse structure and nanometric size range has pulled them to massive exploration as potential carrier for drug delivery to targeted regions. The chemistry of dendrimers offers several modes for incorporation of drugs. Most commonly, drug is linked either covalently or noncovalently to dendrimers. A drug can be noncovalently introduced into dendrimer by simple encapsulation method that is mostly used to enhance solubilization of lipophilic drugs in aqueous media. Charged drugs such as DNA, RNA, or siRNA can also be incorporated into dendrimers through noncovalent electrostatic interactions. Thus, drug can be conjugated in this manner to both the internal and external regions of dendrimer. Covalent incorporation involves formation of stable bonds between drug and dendrimers [39].

Recent research is focused on development of synthetic carriers for delivery of genetic material with low cytotoxicity, highly efficient delivery, and minimal lysosomal degradation [40]. Gene delivery using polyamidoamine (PAMAM) dendrimers has been studied by Haensler and Szoka. Covalent linking of dendrimer with GALA peptide resulted in improved transfection efficiency [41]. Polypropylene imine (PPI) dendrimers enjoying low generations have also shown capacity as DNA carrier for gene transfection with lower cytotoxic potential [42]. Dendrimers have also been explored for delivery of chemotherapeutic agents. Quintana and coworkers have developed PAMAM dendrimers composed of ethylenediamine core. Methotrexate along with targeting ligand and fluorescein was covalently attached to dendritic surface. Experimental data confirmed highly specific binding with KB cell line with 100% improved cytotoxic response as compared to free drug [43]. In another study, siRNA was incorporated in PPI dendrimer that was stabilized using cross-linker to cage the preformed siRNA-dendrimer nanoparticle. PEG layer was applied over this nanostructure that further utilized luteinizing hormone releasing hormone (LHRH) to guide siRNA-loaded nanoparticles to tumor cells. *In-vivo* studies suggested highly specific tumor targeting with improved accumulation of siRNA in cytoplasm of cells and effective gene silencing [44].

Dendritic structures have also inspired boron neutron capture therapy for tumor targeting. To kill tumor cells, it is necessary for ^{10}B to reach intracellular concentration of at least 10^9 atoms/cell. This tumor-specific delivery at desired concentrations has been achieved through use of boronated antibodies. Epidermal growth factor receptors (EGFR) that are overexpressed at surface of glioma cells have been targeted by ^{10}B PAMAM dendrimers. Dendrimers after being covalently linked to epidermal growth factor were effectively internalized by endocytosis with substantial accumulation of ^{10}B in lysosomes of cells *in vitro* [45]. However, *in-vivo* studies demonstrated uptake of boron carriers by the liver and less level of accumulation in C6 glioma cells. To address uptake of boronated dendritic conjugates by the liver, scientists have exploited the steric effect provided by polyethylene oxide (PEO) chains. Such PEO-shielded boronated PAMAM dendrimers showed lesser uptake of conjugate by the liver. However, uptake of PEO-shielded dendritic conjugates by liver was increased with an increase in the number of PEO chains [46].

Exploration of dendrimers in photodynamic therapy (PDT) has also captured great interest. Therapy employs a photosensitizing agent that upon exposure to light of specific wavelength causes irreversible photo-chemical or photo-biological damage to tumor cells. Dendrimers on suitable peripheral functionalization can be promising carrier for photosensitizers. Eighteen ALA (5-aminolevulinic acid) units have been conjugated with dendrimer through amide linkage. These ALA-conjugated dendrimers exhibited increased cellular level of protoporphyrin IX (PIX) and thus showed increased cytotoxicity on exposure of radiations in PAM 212 tumorigenic cell lines [47]. Because of increased tissue permeability to near IR or IR light, the photodynamic system with high absorbance at longer wavelength is extremely attractive. To exploit this feature, aluminum-phthalocyanines polymer conjugates have been designed with the maximum absorption observed at 675 nm [48]. A two-photon approach also has great potential to target deeper tissues with near IR laser. Multivalent character of dendrimers has the capacity to accommodate several two-photon absorbing moieties to porphyrin core. Excitation of chromophores at 780 nm resulted in generation of increased singlet oxygen luminescence [49].

4.2. Semiconductor polymer dots

Semiconducting polymer dots (Pdots), also described as organic nanodots or conjugated polymeric nanoparticles (CPNs), have emerged as promising fluorescent probes due to their exceptional brightness, high quantum yield, nonblinking, photo-stability, and faster emission rate. Pdots, particularly, refer to small semiconducting polymeric nanoparticles and have shown remarkable conduction properties due to the presence of highly delocalized π-conjugated backbone [50]. Pdots prepared by miniemulsion method usually produced polymeric particles with size ranging from 40 to 500 nm depending on nature of polymer and concentration of surfactant. Reprecipitation method yields Pdots in the range of 5–30 nm. Size usually can be modified depending on biological application; however, most bioimaging and assays require smaller nanoparticle. Brightness and photo-stability of fluorescent Pdots appear to increase with size increment but have also exhibited higher steric hindrance, decreasing their target specificity and binding affinity [51]. These carriers have widely investigated for their outstanding potential for bioimaging and biosensing both *in vitro* and *in vivo*. Major advantage lies in lesser cytotoxicity as was observed in the case of inorganic nanocrystals or quantum dots (Qdots) that were also observed to be associated with genotoxic and epigenetic effects in mammalian cells even at minute concentrations [52].

Biological applications of fluorescent probes can be controlled by manipulating surface chemistry. Usually, aqueous solubility is the primary requirement for these particles to perform biological functions efficiently. Such modifications have been carried out by incorporating charged molecules in polymer side chains [53]. Current research has much interest in development of various multifunctional Pdots that offer a wide range of biological applications due to easy preparation and diverse chemical dynamics. Conjugated polymers on the basis of varying structure of backbone can be distinguished into four major categories including poly-(fluorine), poly-(p-phenylene vinylene), poly-(p-phenylene ethynylene), and poly-(thiophene). These polymeric backbones can be further functionalized to incorporate desired characteristics [54]. Wang and coworkers have developed water-soluble conjugated polymer (polythiophene) with tyrosin kinase inhibitor (lapatinib)-modified side chains for plasma membrane imaging by targeting intracellular regions of transmembrane proteins [55]. Scientists have prepared conjugated polymer nanoparticles for both drug delivery and cell imaging together via exploiting electrostatic interactions among cationic conjugated polymers and anionic functionalities. Doxorubicin was delivered to target cancer cells by conjugating it with cationic fluorescent PFO and anionic poly-(L-glutamic acid) that allowed to monitor drug release through 'turn on' fluorescent signal generated by PFO [56].

Apart from cellular imaging, Pdots have also been investigated for delivery of DNA and siRNA. It has been found that nucleic acid carrying a negative charge can be easily incorporated into positively charged semiconductor Pdots. Silva and coworkers have demonstrated the delivery of siRNA using fluorescent CPNs for posttranscriptional gene silencing in plant protoplast without any significant impact on cellular viability in 72 h. They also explained the delivery of siRNA to specifically targeted genes in NTCesA-1 pathway associated with cellulose biosynthesis using CPNs [57]. Moon and associates have developed loosely aggregated CPNs for delivery of siRNA for transfection into HELA cells. siRNA-loaded CPNs caused downregulation of actin b protein with a transfection efficiency of 94% [58].

Scientists have also investigated the role of conjugated polymers for their antimicrobial potential. Cationic, light-absorbing, conjugated polyelectrolytes were studied for their activity against Gram-positive bacterial spores and Gram-negative bacterial strains. The study suggested that conjugated poly-electrolytes formed surface coating on both bacterial types and caused light-induced bactericidal activity [59]. Electrostatic interactions between negatively charged cell surfaces and oppositely charged markers have also been exploited against microbial and cancerous cells. Cationic CPNs have been designed through electrostatic interaction between positively charged PBF and negatively charged SDPA (disodium salt 3,3′-dithiodipropionic acid). These nanoparticles on photoexcitation by white light sensitized production of reactive oxygen species that effectively killed surrounding tumor and bacterial cells along with fluorescent imaging of cellular uptake of these particles [60]. Electrostatic interactions have also been exploited for delivery of doxorubicin through multifunctional CPNs. CPNs (50 nm approx.) with excellent photo-stability and quantum yield but lower cytotoxicity have been prepared by combination of cationic PFO and anionic poly(L-glutamic acid) followed by conjugation with doxorubicin. This carrier offered targeted release of drug in cancer cells along with concurrent examination of drug release via self-luminescence activity [56].

4.3. Carbon dots

Carbon dots (CDs), also known as carbon nanoparticles or carbon quantum dots, are quasi-spherical fluorescent nanoparticles, gaining excessive attention because of unique optical nature, biocompatibility, low cytotoxicity, and simplistic synthesis [61]. These particles were accidently discovered while electrophoretic purification of single-walled carbon nanotubes (SWCNTs) synthesized using arc discharge process. CDs are usually defined as zero-dimensional particles with size range lying around 10 nm. Various synthetic approaches have been investigated for preparation of CDs with efficient photoluminescence, longer wavelength, and multicolor tunable emission [62]. Several types of carbon materials have been engaged to prepare CDs including graphite, activated carbon, carbon nanotubes (CNTs), and nano-diamond using top-down approach [63]. Bottom-up approach has employed citrate, biomolecules, and polymer-silica nanocomposites to prepare CDs using a variety of reaction conditions [64]. CDs have been addressed as safe and biocompatible substitutes to quantum dots that offer better brightness, photo-stability, and lower cytotoxicity both *in vitro* and *in vivo* [65].

Fluorescent CDs have expressed great potential in the field of biosensing, imaging, and photodynamic therapy as well as gene and drug delivery. CDs can be employed for *in-vitro* and *in-vivo* cell imaging using both one- and two-photon excitations. Yang and coworkers have demonstrated biomolecule surface-modified fluorescent carbon dots for *in-vivo* cell imaging along with good biocompatibility and less cytotoxicity [66]. Fluorescent CDs with surface modified with PEG were also studied for *in-vivo* biocompatibility and cytotoxicity through fluorescence imaging [67]. Luo and coworkers have extensively reviewed the optical imaging of carbon dots both *in vitro* and *in vivo* [65]. Various functionalized CDs have been studied for fluorescent imaging of plasma membrane and cytoplasm of COS7 cells, BGC823 cells, MG-63 cells, A549 cells, and HEPG-2 cells [68]. Scientists have also demonstrated uptake of CDs by endosomes and lysosomes in fluorescent imaging of HELA cells [69]. Besides these investigations, some studies have reported distribution of CDs in entire cell including nucleus [70]. CDs have also been explored for cellular imaging and labeling of *E. coli* [63].

CDs have also been investigated as biosensors in various research studies. Fluorescent carbon dots when conjugated with *N*-(2-aminoethyl)-*N, N, N*-tris (pyridin-2-yl methyl) ethane-1, 2-diamine have been studied to detect intracellular Cu^{+2} ions with greater specificity and stability [71]. In another study, fluorescent CDs have been used for detection of metal ions. Scientists have prepared carbon dots from citric acid as a carbon source in the presence of PEI for intracellular imaging and detection of Cu^{+2} ions [72]. Besides metal ion detection, COOH- or OH-functionalized CDs have been used as a receptor to detect change in hydrogen ion concentration. This fluorescent C dot probe has been successfully investigated to detect change in pH of 6–8 range in A549 and LLC-MK2 cells [73]. CDs have been studied for detection of glucose as its transport is associated with certain anomalies such as diabetes and cancer [74].

Scientists have also demonstrated use of CDs for detection of DNA. ssDNA was immobilized on CDs that can get hybridized with required complementary DNA molecule to form dsDNA followed by desorption from CDs and quantification of fluorescence [75]. CDs-dsDNA complex has also been investigated to detect histones. The strong interaction between DNA and histone causing the detachment of DNA from CD that turned on the signal for native fluorescence of CD [76]. CDs conjugated with gold and silver nanostructures have been explored as electro-chemiluminescence (ECL) immuno-sensing devices for detection of prostate-specific antigen (PSA) [77]. CDs have also been conjugated with chlorin e6 (Ce6) photosensitizer for efficient intracellular transport of photosensitizer, longer circulation time, and homing ability in tumor cells. These conjugates revealed excellent stability, biocompatibility with least cytotoxicity and exhibited tremendous bioimaging and homing ability in subcutaneous MGC-803 xenografts in nude mice [78].

Another therapeutic application associated with CDs is gene and drug delivery to targeted cells. pH-responsive, COOH-functionalized CDs caped on surface of mesoporous silica nanoparticles (MSPs) have been studied for intracellular tracking and delivery of doxorubicin with strong luminescence and low cytotoxicity both *in vitro* and *in vivo* [79]. CDs-conjugated mesoporous silica nanoparticles capped with PEG have been investigate for tracking controlled release of doxorubicin through quantifiable fluorescent intensity in HELA cells [80]. In another study, hollow CDs have been prepared from bovine serum albumin for pH-dependent delivery of doxorubicin and its rapid intracellular uptake. Such functionalized hollow CDs have been regarded suitable for bioimaging and targeted drug delivery [81]. Quinolone-conjugated fluorescent CDs have also been explored for *in-vitro* cellular imaging and delivery of drug to cancer cells [82].

4.4. Quantum dots

Quantum dots (Qdots) are inorganic, semiconductor, fluorescent nanostructures composed of II–IV or III–V group elements. They are crystal structures with size smaller than excitation Bohr radius (few nanometers), and these physical dimensions are controllable by time, temperature, and molecules (ligands) used in their synthesis [83]. Qdots in the range of 2–6 nm are of especial interest due to resemblance of their dimensions with biomolecules and have also shown to display strong dimension-dependent electrical and optical characters. Other distinct features include necessity of few Qdots to generate a detectable signal and minimal photo-bleaching property [84]. The idea of quantum confinement is responsible for unique optical and electronic characteristic of Qdots. Both group II–IV and III–V Qdots have been synthesized with relatively lower quantum yield and greater size difference. Higher quantum yield and better luminescence were observed when CdSe core was capped on surface with ZnS or CdS (higher band gap) [85].

The optical character of Qdots has been associated with the interactions among electrons, holes, and surrounding environment. Qdots undergo absorption of photon when excitation energy surpasses band gap where electrons jump from valence band toward conduction band. The presence of multiple electronic states at elevated energy level offers excitation at relatively lower wavelengths across UV-visible spectra. Emission wavelength can be tuned among the region of blue and near infrared (NIR) wavelength by manipulating size and composition of Qdots. This feature allows simultaneous excitation of multicolor Qdots with single light source that makes them excellent candidate for biological application. Bioconjugation and functionalization of Qdots have increased the spectrum of their activities [36]. Qdots have been widely investigated for *in-vitro* and *in-vivo* imaging at molecular and cellular levels, to study intracellular trafficking as well as tumor targeting [86]. Quantum dots have been studied in immunofluorescence assays for detection of biological molecules and labeling of tissues and cells. NIR fluorescent nanoprobes conjugated with copolymer grafts of poly(L-lysine) and methoxy-polyethylene glycol succinate for *in-vivo* imaging of tumor related lysosomal protease activity. These probes successfully detected small-sized solid tumors with higher NIR signals and to examine specific enzyme activity [87]. Qdots have also explored to study the modifications in erythrocyte membranes caused by plasmodium invasion in malaria via immuno-cytochemical studies [88]. Jaiswal and coworkers have demonstrated multicolor imaging of Qdots-labeled live cells. They explained two approaches for cell labeling; either through intracellular uptake of Qdots by endocytic mechanism or use of antibody-conjugated quantum dots specific to cell surface proteins [89]. Parak and associates have used colloidal Qdots to study metastatic potential of cancer cells due to their photochemical stable nature and to study the mechanism of motility and migration of cancer cells. Uptake of nanocrystals was explained to occur through pinocytosis and phagocytosis [90].

Qdots have also been explored to prevent their nonspecific uptake by RES. Molecular markers expressed by blood vessels have been exploited to target nanocarriers toward specific tissues or organs. This strategy has been employed to target lung tumor cells using functionalized Qdots in mice [91]. Surface of quantum dots has been functionalized with COOH, NH2, and streptavidin that was further derivitized using PEG. PEG-conjugated Qdots decreased nonspecific uptake by RES, while COOH- and NH2-functionalized Qdots without PEG showed improved intracellular uptake among various cell types [92]. Qdots have also been explored for gene delivery and gene silencing. Sponge proton-coated Qdot-siRNA has been studied to improve gene silencing efficiency and reduced cytotoxicity in MDA-MB231 cells. These nanocarriers also allowed intracellular tracking and localization of siRNA delivery and transfection [93]. In another study, siRNA transfection was performed using Qdots. siRNA-Qdots exhibited greater photo-stability and tunable optical characteristics. This method was developed to observe the function of T-cadherin in intercellular communication [94].

Chitosan-folate-encapsulated ZnO Qdots have been prepared for delivery of anticancer agent doxorubicin with enhanced and longer photo-stability of Qdots. This nanocarrier showed an initial rapid release followed by controlled liberation of drug [95]. Doxorubicin-loaded, immuno-liposome-based quantum dots were modified with HER2scFv for targeted delivery of drug to SKB-3 and MCF-7 cells with overexpressed HER2. These Qdot-IL conjugates exhibited receptor-dependent endocytosis in target cells but not in control MFC-7 cells. They also showed longer circulation of Qdots, and their localization in tumor models was confirmed by florescence imaging [96]. Cadmium telluride-incorporated Qdots with PEI functionalization for tracking of plasmid DNA in mice were designed. After intravenous injection, these structures showed rapid accumulation in the lungs, spleen, and liver.

PEG functionalization caused improved circulation time and rapid accumulation in cancer cells [97].

4.5. Magnetic nanocarriers

Magnetic nanoparticles (MNPs) are one of other fascinating elements of nanotechnology. Their nanometric dimension, biocompatibility, nontoxicity, and surplus accumulation in targeted cells or tissues justify intensive research in this subject matter. MNPs are mostly composed of ferromagnetic material such as ferrous or ferric oxide core with limited use of cobalt and nickel [98]. Magnetic properties are associated with movement of subatomic particles including electrons, holes, protons, and positive-/negative-charged ions. These materials respond to external stimulus of magnetic field and orient themselves according to magnetic moment. This magnetic behavior has been exploited for both *in-vitro* and *in-vivo* biomedical applications [99]. Magnetic nanoparticles have also been suggested for labeling cells in tissue engineering as they can be easily handled using magnets. Streptavidin-functionalized paramagnetic particles in combination with antibodies have been investigated for magnetic field-guided retroviral infection *in vitro* [100].

Magnetic nanoparticles have the ability to cause ablation of tumor cells via generation of heat. AC magnetic field causes the magnetic particles dispersed in target cells or tissues to get heated. This heat is rapidly disseminated to diseased cells, and if 42°C (therapeutic temperature threshold) can be maintained for 30 min, tumor cells get destroyed. However, this thermal ablation may be associated with undesirable concurrent killing of healthy cells [101]. Hase and coworkers have used ferromagnetic heating in combination of hepatic arterial embolization to study heat induction of ferromagnetic implants on VX2 hepatic cancer in rabbits. Results indicated extensive degeneration of tumor cells suggesting a suitable therapeutic strategy for localized hepatic carcinomas with little damage to healthy parenchyma of the liver because of selective heat induction [102].

Various functionalized magnetic nanocarriers have been investigated for targeted delivery of therapeutic agents. Magnetic drug carriers were designed either by using a magnetic core with surface coated with polymer or magnetic particles precipitated within porous polymeric composite. Such modifications have been studied to protect magnetic particle from harsh physiological vicinity and also to guide the drug carrier to desired location. Magnetic field-guided uncharged magnetic nanoparticles have been investigated for intracerebral targeting of rat glioma-2 in male (Fisher 344) rats. These magnetic nanoparticles (10–20 nm) exhibited greater uptake in brain tumor cells as compared to larger size (1 μm) magnetic particles [103]. In another study, iron oxide core was coated with oleic acid and subsequent coat of PEG-oleic acid for sustained release of doxorubicin and as MRI contrast. These modified magnetic nanoparticles were further conjugated with antibodies for active targeting of MFC-7 cells. These MNPs showed better MRI contrast with longer circulation time. They exhibited sustained release of drug with enhanced antiproliferative effect [104]. Doxorubicin-loaded monodisperse mesoporous single crystal iron oxide nanoparticles have also been developed as a promising carrier with improved drug loading and delivery [105].

5. Conclusion

Multifunctional nanocarriers offer a wide spectrum of biological applications exploiting both extracellular and intracellular barriers. These polymeric nanostructures have successfully improved the efficacy and safety of molecules delivered for various diagnostic and therapeutic purposes. Such nanocarriers have propounded unique physicochemical properties that have overall augmented the pharmacokinetic and pharmacodynamics parameters of drugs owing to versatility in their dimensions and surface functionalization. Bioavailability of many drug molecules that was compromised due to uptake by RES has been enhanced by exploiting these nanodevices. They have also offered long circulation time with release of drug molecules in a controlled or sustained manner with substantially fewer adverse effects. Nanocarriers have also shown exceptional promise in cellular imaging and diagnosis. By using various functionalization techniques, fluorescent probes have been directed to target tissues and cells to study site-specific delivery as well as intracellular trafficking of targeted molecules. Thus, they have been exploited to perform dual role of cell imaging along with drug delivery. Nanocarriers have also been successfully employed for gene transfection and gene silencing as well as *in-vitro* and *in-vivo* detection of biological molecules. Most recent therapeutic strategies under research seem substantially captivated in various dot structures for improved delivery of therapeutic agents, and the same is the case for magnetic nanoparticles that also have offered incredibly assuring results. However, much work is yet to be accomplished to prepare a successful commercial candidate with an ultimate therapeutic spectrum. Critical *in-vivo* cytotoxic behavior of these nanocarriers and untoward effects on normal physiological processes still requires intensive exploration. Some drug-loaded coated nanoparticles have been subjected to preliminary human trials after display of promising outcomes in animal studies but will even so require a long while for appearance in clinical market.

Conflict of interest

There is no conflict of interests among authors.

Author details

Maria Hassan Kiani[1], Masoom Yasinzai[2] and Gul Shahnaz[1]*

*Address all correspondence to: gshahnaz@qau.edu.pk

1 Department of Pharmacy, Faculty of Biological Sciences, Quaid-i-Azam University, Islamabad, Pakistan

2 Centre for Interdisciplinary Research in Basic Sciences, International Islamic University, Islamabad, Pakistan

References

[1] Cho K et al. Therapeutic nanoparticles for drug delivery in cancer. Clinical Cancer Research. 2008;**14**(5):1310-1316

[2] Bareford LM, Swaan PW. Endocytic mechanisms for targeted drug delivery. Advanced Drug Delivery Reviews. 2007;**59**(8):748-758

[3] Senior JH. Fate and behavior of liposomes in vivo: A review of controlling factors. Critical Reviews in Therapeutic Drug Carrier Systems. 1987;**3**(2):123-193

[4] Gref R et al. The controlled intravenous delivery of drugs using PEG-coated sterically stabilized nanospheres. Advanced Drug Delivery Reviews. 2012;**64**(Supplement):316-326

[5] Singh R, Lillard JW. Nanoparticle-based targeted drug delivery. Experimental and Molecular Pathology. 2009;**86**(3):215-223

[6] Torchilin VP. Recent approaches to intracellular delivery of drugs and DNA and organelle targeting. Annual Review of Biomedical Engineering. 2006;**8**(1):343-375

[7] Varga CM, Wickham TJ, Lauffenburger DA. Receptor-mediated targeting of gene delivery vectors: Insights from molecular mechanisms for improved vehicle design. Biotechnology and Bioengineering. 2000;**70**(6):593-605

[8] Wileman T, Harding C, Stahl P. Receptor-mediated endocytosis. Biochemical Journal. 1985;**232**(1):1-14

[9] Nichols BJ, Lippincott-Schwartz J. Endocytosis without clathrin coats. Trends in Cell Biology. 2001;**11**(10):406-412

[10] Stahl P, Schwartz AL. Receptor-mediated endocytosis. Journal of Clinical Investigation. 1986;**77**(3):657-662

[11] Jois SD et al. Solution structure of a cyclic RGD peptide that inhibits platelet aggregation. Journal of Biomolecular Structure and Dynamics. 1996;**14**(1):1-11

[12] Tejo BA et al. Structural modifications of ICAM-1 cyclic peptides to improve the activity to inhibit heterotypic adhesion of T cells. Chemical Biology & Drug Design. 2008;**72**(1):27-33

[13] Triantafilou K, Takada Y, Triantafilou M. Mechanisms of integrin-mediated virus attachment and internalization process. Critical Reviews in Immunology. 2001;**21**(4):311-322

[14] Sandvig K, van Deurs B. Endocytosis without clathrin: A minireview. Cell Biology International Reports. 1991;**15**(1):3-8

[15] Bathori G, Cervenak L, Karadi I. Caveolae--an alternative endocytotic pathway for targeted drug delivery. Critical Reviews in Therapeutic Drug Carrier Systems. 2004;**21**(2): 67-95

[16] Kurzchalia TV, Partan RG. Membrane microdomains and caveolae. Current Opinion in Cell Biology. 1999;**11**(4):424-431

[17] Kerr MC, Teasdale RD. Defining macropinocytosis. Traffic. 2009;**10**(4):364-371

[18] Stromhaug PE et al. Differences between fluid-phase endocytosis (pinocytosis) and receptor-mediated endocytosis in isolated rat hepatocytes. European Journal Cell Biology. 1997;**73**(1):28-39

[19] Mitra A et al. Technetium-99 m-labeled N-(2-hydroxypropyl) methacrylamide copolymers: Synthesis, characterization, and in vivo biodistribution. Pharmaceutical Research. 2004;**21**(7):1153-1159

[20] Moghimi SM, Hunter AC, Murray JC. Long-circulating and target-specific nanoparticles: Theory to practice. Pharmacological Reviews. 2001;**53**(2):283-318

[21] Soppimath KS et al. Biodegradable polymeric nanoparticles as drug delivery devices. Journal of Controlled Release. 2001;**70**(1):1-20

[22] Friberg SE. A review of: "Colloid carriers for controlled drug delivery and targeting:" modification, characterization and in vivo distribution, R.H.Müller, ed., CRC Press, Boca Raton, FL, 1991. Journal of Dispersion Science and Technology. 1995;**16**(5):395-395

[23] Müller RH, Wallis KH. Surface modification of i.v. injectable biodegradable nanoparticles with poloxamer polymers and poloxamine 908. International Journal of Pharmaceutics. 1993;**89**(1):25-31

[24] Lockman P et al. Nanoparticle technology for drug delivery across the blood-brain barrier. Drug Development and Industrial Pharmacy. 2002;**28**(1):1-13

[25] Olivier JC et al. Indirect evidence that drug brain targeting using polysorbate 80-coated polybutylcyanoacrylate nanoparticles is related to toxicity. Pharmaceutical Research. 1999;**16**(12):1836-1842

[26] Fenart L et al. Evaluation of effect of charge and lipid coating on ability of 60-nm nanoparticles to cross an in vitro model of the blood-brain barrier. Journal of Pharmacology and Experimental Therapeutics. 1999;**291**(3):1017-1022

[27] Couvreur P, Puisieux F. Nano- and microparticles for the delivery of polypeptides and proteins. Advanced Drug Delivery Reviews. 1993;**10**(2):141-162

[28] Manuela Gaspar M et al. Formulation of l-asparaginase-loaded poly(lactide-co-glycolide) nanoparticles: Influence of polymer properties on enzyme loading, activity and in vitro release. Journal of Controlled Release. 1998;**52**(1):53-62

[29] Al Khouri Fallouh N et al. Development of a new process for the manufacture of polyisobutylcyanoacrylate nanocapsules. International Journal of Pharmaceutics. 1986;**28**(2): 125-132

[30] Leroux J-C et al. Biodegradable nanoparticles — From sustained release formulations to improved site specific drug delivery. Journal of Controlled Release. 1996;**39**(2):339-350

[31] Damge C et al. New approach for oral administration of insulin with polyalkylcyanoacrylate nanocapsules as drug carrier. Diabetes. 1988;**37**(2):246-251

[32] Musumeci T et al. PLA/PLGA nanoparticles for sustained release of docetaxel. International Journal of Pharmaceutics. 2006;**325**(1):172-179

[33] Kojima C et al. Synthesis of polyamidoamine dendrimers having poly(ethylene glycol) grafts and their ability to encapsulate anticancer drugs. Bioconjugate Chemistry. 2000;**11**(6):910-917

[34] Mu L, Feng S-S. PLGA/TPGS nanoparticles for controlled release of paclitaxel: Effects of the emulsifier and drug loading ratio. Pharmaceutical Research. 2003;**20**(11):1864-1872

[35] Torchilin VP. Liposomes as targetable drug carriers. Critical Reviews in Therapeutic Drug Carrier Systems. 1985;**2**(1):65-115

[36] Anurogo D, Parikesit AA, Ikrar T. Bionanomedicine: A "panacea" in medicine? Makara Journal of Health Research. 2017;**21**(2):42-48

[37] Liu M, Fréchet JMJ. Designing dendrimers for drug delivery. Pharmaceutical Science and Technology Today. 1999;**2**(10):393-401

[38] Aulenta F, Hayes W, Rannard S. Dendrimers: A new class of nanoscopic containers and delivery devices. European Polymer Journal. 2003;**39**(9):1741-1771

[39] Turrin C-O, Caminade A-M. Dendrimer conjugates for drug delivery. In: Dendrimers. United Kingdom: John Wiley & Sons, Ltd; 2011. pp. 437-461

[40] Uhrich K. Hyperbranched polymers for drug delivery. Trends in Polymer Science. 1997; **5**(12):388-393

[41] Haensler J, Szoka FC. Polyamidoamine cascade polymers mediate efficient transfection of cells in culture. Bioconjugate Chemistry. 1993;**4**(5):372-379

[42] Hollins AJ et al. Evaluation of generation 2 and 3 poly(propylenimine) dendrimers for the potential cellular delivery of antisense oligonucleotides targeting the epidermal growth factor receptor. Pharmaceutical Research. 2004;**21**(3):458-466

[43] Quintana A et al. Design and function of a dendrimer-based therapeutic nanodevice targeted to tumor cells through the folate receptor. Pharmaceutical Research. 2002; **19**(9):1310-1316

[44] Taratula O et al. Surface-engineered targeted PPI dendrimer for efficient intracellular and intratumoral siRNA delivery. Journal of Controlled Release. 2009;**140**(3):284-293

[45] Capala J et al. Boronated epidermal growth factor as a potential targeting agent for boron neutron capture therapy of brain tumors. Bioconjugate Chemistry. 1996;**7**(1):7-15

[46] Shukla S et al. Synthesis and biological evaluation of folate receptor-targeted boronated PAMAM dendrimers as potential agents for neutron capture therapy. Bioconjugate Chemistry. 2003;**14**(1):158-167

[47] Battah SH et al. Synthesis and biological studies of 5-aminolevulinic acid containing dendrimers for photodynamic therapy. Bioconjugate Chemistry. 2001;**12**(6):980-988

[48] Brasseur N et al. Water-soluble aluminium phthalocyanine–polymer conjugates for PDT: Photodynamic activities and pharmacokinetics in tumour-bearing mice. British Journal of Cancer. 1999;**80**:1533

[49] Dichtel WR et al. Singlet oxygen generation via two-photon excited FRET. Journal of the American Chemical Society. 2004;**126**(17):5380-5381

[50] Feng L et al. Conjugated polymer nanoparticles: Preparation, properties, functionalization and biological applications. Chemical Society Reviews. 2013;**42**(16):6620-6633

[51] Wu C, Chiu DT. Highly fluorescent semiconducting polymer dots for biology and medicine. Angewandte Chemie International Edition. 2013;**52**(11):3086-3109

[52] Winnik FM, Maysinger D. Quantum dot cytotoxicity and ways to reduce it. Accounts of Chemical Research. 2013;**46**(3):672-680

[53] Thomas SW, Joly GD, Swager TM. Chemical sensors based on amplifying fluorescent conjugated polymers. Chemical Reviews. 2007;**107**(4):1339-1386

[54] Liu B et al. Shape-adaptable water-soluble conjugated polymers. Journal of the American Chemical Society. 2003;**125**(44):13306-13307

[55] Wang B et al. Synthesis of a new conjugated polymer for cell membrane imaging by using an intracellular targeting strategy. Polymer Chemistry. 2013;**4**(20):5212-5215

[56] Feng X et al. Conjugated polymer nanoparticles for drug delivery and imaging. ACS Applied Materials & Interfaces. 2010;**2**(8):2429-2435

[57] Silva AT et al. Conjugated polymer nanoparticles for effective siRNA delivery to tobacco BY-2 protoplasts. BMC Plant Biology. 2010;**10**(1):291

[58] Moon JH et al. Conjugated polymer nanoparticles for small interfering RNA delivery. Chemical Communications. 2011;**47**(29):8370-8372

[59] Lu L et al. Biocidal activity of a light-absorbing fluorescent conjugated polyelectrolyte. Langmuir. 2005;**21**(22):10154-10159

[60] Chong H et al. Conjugated polymer nanoparticles for light-activated anticancer and antibacterial activity with imaging capability. Langmuir. 2012;**28**(4):2091-2098

[61] Sun X, Lei Y. Fluorescent carbon dots and their sensing applications. TrAC Trends in Analytical Chemistry. 2017;**89**(Supplement C):163-180

[62] Wu ZL, Liu ZX, Yuan YH. Carbon dots: Materials, synthesis, properties and approaches to long-wavelength and multicolor emission. Journal of Materials Chemistry B. 2017;**5**(21):3794-3809

[63] Sun Y-P et al. Quantum-sized carbon dots for bright and colorful photoluminescence. Journal of the American Chemical Society. 2006;**128**(24):7756-7757

[64] Liu H, Ye T, Mao C. Fluorescent carbon nanoparticles derived from candle soot. Angewandte Chemie International Edition. 2007;**46**(34):6473-6475

[65] Luo PG et al. Carbon "quantum" dots for optical bioimaging. Journal of Materials Chemistry B. 2013;**1**(16):2116-2127

[66] Yang S-T et al. Carbon dots for optical imaging in vivo. Journal of the American Chemical Society. 2009;**131**(32):11308-11309

[67] Yang S-T et al. Carbon dots as nontoxic and high-performance fluorescence imaging agents. The Journal of Physical Chemistry C. 2009;**113**(42):18110-18114

[68] Wang F et al. Highly luminescent organosilane-functionalized carbon dots. Advanced Functional Materials. 2011;**21**(6):1027-1031

[69] Li N et al. Biodistribution study of carbogenic dots in cells and in vivo for optical imaging. Journal of Nanoparticle Research. 2012;**14**(10):1177

[70] Ray S et al. Fluorescent carbon nanoparticles: Synthesis, characterization, and bioimaging application. The Journal of Physical Chemistry C. 2009;**113**(43):18546-18551

[71] Zhu A et al. Carbon-dot-based dual-emission nanohybrid produces a ratiometric fluorescent sensor for in vivo imaging of cellular copper ions. Angewandte Chemie. 2012; **124**(29):7297-7301

[72] Salinas-Castillo A et al. Carbon dots for copper detection with down and upconversion fluorescent properties as excitation sources. Chemical Communications. 2013; **49**(11):1103-1105

[73] Kong B et al. Carbon dot-based inorganic-organic nanosystem for two-photon imaging and biosensing of pH variation in living cells and tissues. Advanced Materials. 2012; **24**(43):5844-5848

[74] Qu Z-b et al. Boronic acid functionalized graphene quantum dots as a fluorescent probe for selective and sensitive glucose determination in microdialysate. Chemical Communications. 2013;**49**(84):9830-9832

[75] Li H et al. Nucleic acid detection using carbon nanoparticles as a fluorescent sensing platform. Chemical Communications. 2011;**47**(3):961-963

[76] Maiti S, Das K, Das PK. Label-free fluorimetric detection of histone using quaternized carbon dot–DNA nanobiohybrid. Chemical Communications. 2013;**49**(78):8851-8853

[77] Wu L et al. Ultrasensitive electrochemiluminescence immunosensor for tumor marker detection based on nanoporous sliver@ carbon dots as labels. Sensors and Actuators B: Chemical. 2013;**186**:761-767

[78] Huang P et al. Light-triggered theranostics based on photosensitizer-conjugated carbon dots for simultaneous enhanced-fluorescence imaging and photodynamic therapy. Advanced Materials. 2012;**24**(37):5104-5110

[79] Zhou L et al. Luminescent carbon dot-gated nanovehicles for pH-triggered intracellular controlled release and imaging. Langmuir. 2013;**29**(21):6396-6403

[80] Lai C-W et al. Facile synthesis of highly emissive carbon dots from pyrolysis of glycerol; gram scale production of carbon dots/mSiO_2 for cell imaging and drug release. Journal of Materials Chemistry. 2012;**22**(29):14403-14409

[81] Wang Q et al. Hollow luminescent carbon dots for drug delivery. Carbon. 2013;**59**:192-199

[82] Karthik S et al. Photoresponsive quinoline tethered fluorescent carbon dots for regulated anticancer drug delivery. Chemical Communications. 2013;**49**(89):10471-10473

[83] Alivisatos AP et al. Organization of'nanocrystal molecules' using DNA. Nature. 1996; **382**(6592):609

[84] Moras JD et al. Semiconductor clusters, nanocrystals, and quantum dots. Science. 1996; **271**:933

[85] Dabbousi BO et al. (CdSe) ZnS core-shell quantum dots: Synthesis and characterization of a size series of highly luminescent nanocrystallites. The Journal of Physical Chemistry B. 1997;**101**(46):9463-9475

[86] Chan WC, Nie S. Quantum dot bioconjugates for ultrasensitive nonisotopic detection. Science. 1998;**281**(5385):2016-2018

[87] Weissleder R et al. In vivo imaging of tumors with protease-activated near-infrared fluorescent probes. Nature Biotechnology. 1999;**17**:375

[88] Tokumasu F, Dvorak J. Development and application of quantum dots for immunocytochemistry of human erythrocytes. Journal of Microscopy. 2003;**211**(3):256-261

[89] Jaiswal JK et al. Long-term multiple color imaging of live cells using quantum dot bioconjugates. Nature Biotechnology. 2002;**21**:47

[90] Parak WJ et al. Cell motility and metastatic potential studies based on quantum dot imaging of phagokinetic tracks. Advanced Materials. 2002;**14**(12):882-885

[91] Åkerman ME et al. Nanocrystal targeting in vivo. Proceedings of the National Academy of Sciences. 2002;**99**(20):12617-12621

[92] Kelf TA et al. Non-specific cellular uptake of surface-functionalized quantum dots. Nanotechnology. 2010;**21**(28):285105

[93] Yezhelyev MV et al. Proton-sponge coated quantum dots for siRNA delivery and intracellular imaging. Journal of the American Chemical Society. 2008;**130**(28):9006-9012

[94] Chen AA et al. Quantum dots to monitor RNAi delivery and improve gene silencing. Nucleic Acids Research. 2005;**33**(22):e190-e190

[95] Yuan Q, Hein S, Misra RDK. New generation of chitosan-encapsulated ZnO quantum dots loaded with drug: Synthesis, characterization and in vitro drug delivery response. Acta Biomaterialia. 2010;**6**(7):2732-2739

[96] Weng KC et al. Targeted tumor cell internalization and imaging of multifunctional quantum dot-conjugated immunoliposomes in vitro and in vivo. Nano Letters. 2008; **8**(9):2851-2857

[97] Zintchenko A et al. Drug nanocarriers labeled with near-infrared-emitting quantum dots (quantoplexes): Imaging fast dynamics of distribution in living animals. Molecular Therapy. 2009;**17**(11):1849-1856

[98] Ito A et al. Medical application of functionalized magnetic nanoparticles. Journal of Bioscience and Bioengineering. 2005;**100**(1):1-11

[99] Pankhurst QA et al. Applications of magnetic nanoparticles in biomedicine. Journal of Physics D: Applied Physics. 2003;**36**(13):R167

[100] Ito A et al. Construction and harvest of multilayered keratinocyte sheets using magnetite nanoparticles and magnetic force. Tissue Engineering. 2004;**10**(5-6):873-880

[101] Rand R et al. Selective radiofrequency heating of ferrosilicone occluded tissue: A preliminary report. Bulletin of the Los Angeles Neurological Societies. 1976;**41**(4):154

[102] Hase M, Sako M, Hirota S. Experimental study of ferromagnetic induction heating combined with hepatic arterial embolization for treatment of liver tumors. Nihon Igaku Hoshasen Gakkai zasshi. Nippon Acta Radiologica. 1990;**50**(11):1402-1414

[103] Pulfer SK, Ciccotto SL, Gallo JM. Distribution of small magnetic particles in brain tumor-bearing rats. Journal of Neuro-Oncology. 1999;**41**(2):99-105

[104] Yallapu MM et al. Peg-functionalized magnetic nanoparticles for drug delivery and magnetic resonance imaging applications. Pharmaceutical Research. 2010;**27**(11):2283-2295

[105] Guo S et al. Monodisperse mesoporous superparamagnetic single-crystal magnetite nanoparticles for drug delivery. Biomaterials. 2009;**30**(10):1881-1889

Chapter 6

Multifunctional Nanoparticles for Successful Targeted Drug Delivery across the Blood-Brain Barrier

Débora Braga Vieira and Lionel Fernel Gamarra

Additional information is available at the end of the chapter

http://dx.doi.org/10.5772/intechopen.76922

Abstract

The blood-brain barrier (BBB) is the major problem for the treatment of brain diseases because we need to be able to deliver drugs from the vascular system into the central nervous system (CNS). There are no drug therapies for a wide range of CNS diseases and these include neurodegenerative diseases such as Alzheimer's and Parkinson's diseases and cerebral ischemia. Therefore, the focus of this chapter is to discuss how nanoparticles (NPs) can be modified to transport different drug molecules for the treatment of brain diseases. In essence, NPs' surface can be functionalized with molecules such as peptides, antibodies and RNA aptamers and these macromolecules can be attached to the receptors present at the BBB endothelial cell surface, which allows the NPs cross the barrier and subsequently deliver pharmaceuticals to the brain for the therapeutic and/or imaging of neurological disorders. In fact, part of the difficulty in finding an effective treatment for these CNS disorders is that there is not yet an efficient delivery method for drug delivery across the BBB. However, over the last several years, researches have started to understand some of the design rules to efficiently deliver NPs to the brain.

Keywords: blood-brain barrier, multifunctional nanoparticles, Alzheimer's, Parkinson's, cerebral ischemia, stroke

1. Introduction

Technological innovations, referred to as nanomedicine, is an exciting field of applications of nanotechnology to the diagnostic, treatment and/or prevention of traumatic injury or disease of the human body. This field holds the promise to deeply revolutionize the medicine to treatment and therapy areas such as imaging, drug delivery, cell therapy, tissue regeneration and development of new nanomedicine products. Due to its great importance, recent global marketed report expects that the applications of nanotechnology in medicine could reach $528 billion by 2019 [1]. Indeed, a broad range of nanoparticles (NPs) made of various materials (e.g., polymers, dendrimers, gold, silver, lipids, metals, and virus-like particles), differing in their size, architecture and surface properties, has been initially engineered to improve parameters such as the pharmacokinetics and biodistribution of therapeutic molecules and to reduce drugs' toxicity side effects [2]. Additionally, NPs are also useful tools for body or organ imaging [3]. During the past few decades, NPs have been successfully developed as drug, gene and/or imaging delivery vehicles due to their key properties of enhancing water solubility of poorly water-soluble molecules, extending the plasma circulation time and targeting the site of disease, while avoiding nonspecific toxicity effects [4, 5].

In fact, NPs have provided remarkable progress in therapy and diagnostic imaging of several diseases. Since 1990, a high number of nanocarrier formulations have been approved by regulatory authorities for clinical use [6, 7]. There are five different applications of nanomedicine products on the market within healthcare – *in vitro* diagnostics; biomaterials; drug delivery; *in vivo* imaging and active implants [7]. Of these products, the type of NPs that exists on the market is diverse and it includes the following: (i) liposomes (e.g., Ambisome®, Albelcet®, DaunoXome®, Depocyt® and Myocet®); (ii) polymer-coated liposomes (e.g., Doxil® and Lipo-Dox®); (iii) polymeric drugs (e.g., Copaxone®); (iv) polymer-protein conjugates (e.g., Oncospar®, PEG-Intron® and Pegasys®); (v) nanoparticle containing paclitaxel (e.g., Abraxane™), (vi) antibodies (e.g., Avastin™ and Herceptin®) and (vii) antibody conjugates (e.g., Mylotarg®); (viii) aptamer conjugates (e.g., Macugen®); (viii) micelles (e.g., Estrasorb®); among others. These formulations are considered the first generation of nanomedicine, already bringing clinical benefits to patients [8].

Moreover, researches are constantly focusing on the development of NPs that can accumulate and deliver their cargo specifically at the diseased site, and these efforts are bringing important advances toward the development of NP-based targeted drug delivery systems. To increase the specificity of NPs to the targeted area, nanocarriers that can either passively or actively target the unhealthy site have been engineered. In passive targeting, the capacity of NPs to accumulate in the angiogenic site of tumors by the enhanced permeability and retention effect is explored [6, 9]. This strategy is achieved by recovering surface of NPs with some sort of coating with several compounds such as poly(ethylene glycol) (PEG) and poly(phosphoester) (PEEP) [10]. By binding PEG or PEEP to the surface of NPs, there occurs a change in the protein corona populations that adhere to the surface of NPs, reducing drastically the opsonization process of the nanocarriers thus preventing recognition by macrophages and monocytes and rapid clearance of NPs from the blood [10, 11]. Also, the accumulation and cellular uptake of NPs could be further enhanced by conjugating the NPs with molecules such as antibodies, peptides and aptamers that are able to bind to overexpressed receptor or antigens on the surface of targeted cells [12].

More recently, various researchers have been developing NPs able to perform two or more functions for the simultaneous or sequential delivery of single or multiple therapeutic active principles to the required targeted site in the body, overcoming multiple physiological barriers [13]. Multifunctional NPs often have the ability to: (i) encapsulate sufficient amount of drug or therapeutic macromolecules for a sufficient time; (ii) increase residence time in the blood through the use of soluble polymers such as polyethylene glycol (PEG); (iii) increase their accumulation at the desired site in the body by attaching to NPs, surface macromolecules such as antibodies, RNA aptamers and peptides; (iii) respond to several intrinsic or extrinsic stimuli for "on demand" delivery such as abnormal pH, temperature or magnetic and ultrasound fields and (iv) entrap concomitantly an imaging agent to enable the real-time monitoring of their biodistribution, targeted accumulation and/or therapy efficiency [2, 13].

Despite the exciting advances in the discipline of nanotechnology-based approaches, different challenges arise in their efficacy toward the treatment of neurodegenerative diseases. One of the major obstacles that limit the application of NPs for effective delivery of drugs and diagnostic imaging agents to the central nervous system (CNS) is the presence of the blood-brain barrier (BBB) [14]. As a result, new and innovative invasive and noninvasive NPs formulations have been engineered to provide efficacy in crossing the BBB, mainly by the functionalization of NPs' surface with ligands. Invasive strategies show potential and are being explored for efficient NPs' access to the brain. Some examples of invasive strategies are: convention-enhanced delivery, intracerebral or nasal injection and use of implants. With this in mind, it is important to understand the general concept of BBB, mechanisms of transport in and out of the brain and the BBB alterations in pathology.

2. BBB, general concept and the transport of drugs inside the brain

The BBB is a formidable physiological structure that acts as an effective security system for the brain, letting in circulating compounds that this organ needs, but at the same time, these cells have evolved a system of biological pumps and if these pumps recognize molecules that should not be on their way to the brain, they will be pumped right back out into the vascular system [15]. The BBB is primarily composed of brain endothelial cells, which are cells that line microvessels and capillaries in the brain, and these are highly specialized cells that are knitted together very tightly by tight junctions, so there are no gaps between the cells (**Figure 1**). In fact, endothelial cells' tight junctions control the flux of hydrophilic molecules and small lipophilic substances such as water and some gases, respectively, that go through the BBB [15, 16]. Also, the brain endothelial cells are surrounded by a structure known as basal lamina, composed of fibronectin, type IV collagen, heparin sulfate and laminin [16, 17].

Other structures such as neurons, astrocytes, pericytes and extracellular matrix components constitute the neurovascular unit that is also part of the BBB structure (**Figure 1**). Neurons are electrically excitable cells responsible for processing and transmitting information throughout the mind and body. In the nervous system, chemical and electrical signals between neurons occur via synapses, or junctions, that connect these cells [18]. Astrocytes play a key role in providing nutrients to neurons by shuttling them from the blood vessels to neurons themselves; they also help to control the ion concentration in the brain; are part of the repair process that happens after brain injury and help neurons recycle their neurotransmitters [19].

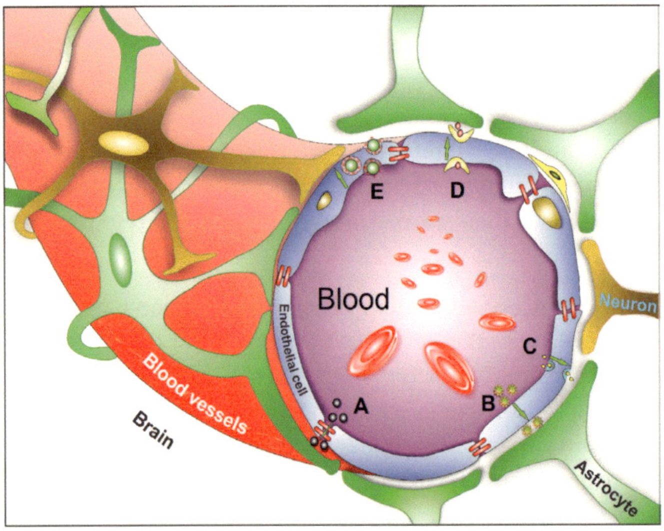

Figure 1. The Blood-Brain Barrier. Schematic cross-sectional representation of the blood brain barrier (BBB) and other components of vascular unit like neurons, astrocytes, pericytes that are essential for the health function of the CNS. Also, depicted in the picture are the BBB mechanism of passage: (A) Water soluble agents; (B) Lipid solid agents; (C) Protein transport; (D) Receptor-mediated transport, and (E) Adsorptive transcytosis.

Pericytes appear to play a key role in BBB endothelial cells barrier formation [20]. Finally, the extracellular matrix occupies 10–20% of brain volume and has a major role in its normal pathology [21]. Therefore, it is the vascular unit that controls permeability and cerebral blood flow throughout the CNS, ensuring physiological CNS functioning.

In **Figure 1**, a schematic overview of the mechanisms of transport through the BBB is depicted. Molecules that present either a high degree of lipophilicity and molecular weight smaller than 500 Da can penetrate the CNS by simple diffusion (**Figure 1A**). However, in the absence of these characteristics, other circulating molecules can cross the BBB by their interaction with specific transport proteins located at the brain endothelial surface. These proteins are classified into two main categories: (i) carrier-mediated transport and (ii) receptor-mediated transport. Carrier-mediated transport (CTM) systems are responsible for the transport of small-drug molecules or small nutrient molecules including monosaccharaides and amino acids with a molecular mass smaller than 600 Da. These molecules can cross the BBB endothelial cells via active transport mediated by specific proteins (**Figure 2C**). The diffusion of molecules from the blood to the brain may be passive or active. For example, the transport of neutral L-amino acids such as leucine, phenylalanine and tyrosine is mediated by the large neutral amino acid transport (LAT1), whereas cationic amino acid transporter (CAT1) mediates the transport of cationic amino acids such as lysine and histidine. Other examples of transporters of polar substances into the brain include the nucleoside transporter (CNT2), the glucose transporter (GLUT1) and the monocarboxylic acid transporter (MCT1) for nucleoside, glucose and carboxylic acids transport, respectively. Moreover, transporters presented at brain endothelial cells' surface are also able to expel endogenous peptides such as Tyr-Pro-Trp-Gly or a multiplicity of drugs from the CNS to the blood are to be mediated, respectively, by peptide

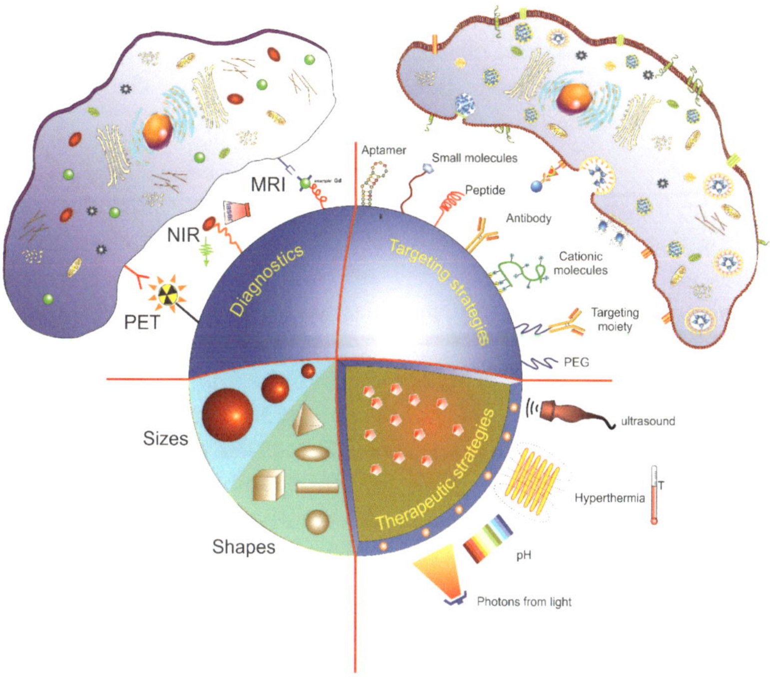

Figure 2. Schematic representation of a drug-loaded, multifunctional, stimuli-responsive NP. The structure of a nanocarrier allows the incorporation of one or multiple therapeutic molecules. These NPs can be found in different sizes and shapes. Increased blood circulation time can be achieved with soluble polymers such as polyethylene glycol (PEG). Nonspecifically target the intended site of action can be achieved by exploring, for example, leaky vessels of tumors. NPs can be actively targeted via the attachment of targeted-specific ligands such as antibody, antibody fragments, aptamers and peptides at their surface. Depending on the kind of application of NPs, various compounds can be added to turn the nanocarrier into a responsive device to a specific stimuli such as temperature, pH or magnetic and ultrasound fields. Imaging or contrast agents such as magnetic resonance imaging (MRI) , near infrared (NIR) and/ or polyethylene terephthalate (PET) compounds can also be incorporated into a single platform to enable imaging and releasing of drugs from NPs.

transport system-1 or P-glycoprotein, via active efflux transport (AET). In fact, if a drug is a substrate of any AET protein, multidrug resistance occurs, and this phenomenon is a great obstacle for therapeutic drug delivery to the CNS.

Chemotherapy agents, natural, synthesized or recombinant peptides and proteins, nucleic acids, monoclonal antibodies and other pharmaceutical breakthroughs do not readily cross the BBB (**Figure 2D**). Nonetheless, there are some specific proteins that the brain needs to function correctly, so they can access the brain by attaching to receptors, which are transported across the barrier and subsequently release into the brain. This mechanism of transport is known as receptor-mediated transport (RMT) and the internalization of these relatively large compounds is done via endocytosis (**Figure 2E**). It is the most studied transport mechanism for drug delivery, since receptor-specific ligands such as peptides and antibodies against receptors that are expressed on brain endothelial cells surface can be attached to the surface of nanoparticles or drugs, enabling their accumulation and internalization by cells of vascular side and, consequently, being transported into the brain. In addition, adsorptive-mediated transport (AMT) is a kind of transport where endocytosis is induced by the binding of cationic substances to the negatively charged plasma membrane of brain endothelial cells interaction. Therefore, due to the electrostatic interaction between the negatively charged membranes, the cationic therapeutic compound takes the AMT to enter the CNS.

This becomes a problem when treating diseases of the brain because we need to be able to deliver drugs from the vascular system into the CNS [22]. Unfortunately, at the moment, there are no drug therapies for a wide range of CNS diseases, and these include neurodegenerative diseases such as Alzheimer's disease (AD) and Parkinson's disease (PD) and cerebral ischemia (or stroke). Therefore, the objective of this chapter is to discuss how NPs can be modified to transport thousands of different drug molecules for the treatment of brain diseases. In essence, NPs for drug delivery into the brain is a method for transporting drug molecules across the BBB using nanocarriers. NPs, surface can be functionalized with molecules such as peptides, antibodies and RNA aptamers, and these macromolecules can be attached to the receptors present at the BBB endothelial cell surface, which allow the NPs across the barrier and subsequently deliver pharmaceuticals to the brain for the therapeutic and/or imaging of neurological disorders [14]. In fact, part of the difficulty in finding an effective treatment for these CNS disorders is that there is not yet an efficient delivery method for drug delivery across the BBB. However, over the last several years, researches have started to understand some of the design rules for efficient delivery of NPs to the brain.

3. *In vitro* approaches to study NPs' transport through the BBB

As mentioned earlier, the BBB is a selective and dynamic barrier restricting the passage of a huge variety of compounds across this barrier, which is essential for the maintenance of homeostasis and functionality of the CNS. Therefore, the BBB is considered the major obstacle for the use of NPs as delivery systems to brain diseases. As shown in **Figure 2**, endothelial cells of the cerebral microvasculature are associated with perivascular cells form the BBB. The functional interaction between endothelial and perivascular cells and their response to injury have led to the concept of the neurovascular unit [15, 17]. Studying the mechanisms of uptake, transport and cytotoxicity of NPs through the BBB is an extremely challenging task *in vivo* because of the technical limitation to access the interface between the vascular system and the brain, since it is estimated that the brain capillary length is about 650 km [23]. To overcome this problem, *in vitro* BBB models have been built to reproduce as precise as possible the major BBB features, allowing investigation of cellular and molecular mechanisms that occur in the barrier; prediction of the transport of compounds across the BBB and performing high-throughput platform to test NPs transport through the barrier for the effective treatment of brain diseases. For example, it was observed that NPs can reach the capillaries into the brain of rats or mice 30 m after intravenous injection and, up to 5 h after NPs administration, they could go through the barrier, decreasing afterward [24–29]. These studies of NPs across the brain tissue are in line with *in vitro* BBB models data reported [30, 31]. In addition, it was observed that *in vitro* BBB model facilitates the manipulation of some parameters that affects the barrier such as aglycemia, hypoxia, among others [32]. For decades, two-dimensional or three-dimensional *in vitro* models of BBB have been developed by cultivating either as a monolayer or in cocultivation with mouse brain microvascular endothelial cells and murine or human endothelial cells with pericytes or astrocytes or glial tissue among others in a way that mimics the barrier under physiological or pathological conditions such as Alzheimer's and Parkinson's diseases or stroke [33–37]. Models of BBB based on stem cells are also reported in the literature [38, 39]. Moreover, by taking permeability measurements on the cultured cells, it is possible to test the physiological relevance of the developed model. In addition, experiments such as gene expression analysis using real-time polymerase chain reaction (PCR), permeability analysis [40, 41] and immunocytochemistry can also be used to validate the BBB model obtained. Although we are still not able to make this platform available both in academic and industry setting, this kind of technology has been showing the importance of considering *in vitro* data together with *in vivo* studies to understand the transport process of NPs into the brain.

4. Other barriers that limit effective drug delivery into the brain

In addition, the BBB is not the only physiological barrier for drug delivery to the brain. If we consider the anatomic aspects of our body, the brain and the spinal cord are completely cushioned and protected by the cerebrospinal fluid (CSF) [42, 43]. This fluid is also responsible for carrying nutrients to and waste products away from the brain. The great majority of CSF is produced within ventricular areas of the brain, as a result of the specialized tissue known as choroid plexus. The choroid plexus is located in each of the four ventricles within the brain area: two lateral ventricles, and the third and fourth ventricles. Here, it is important to clarify that the cells of the choroid plexus do not produce the CSF; instead, this fluid is a filtrate of the blood that is performed by the highly specialized cells of choroid plexus known as cuboidal epithelial cells. Cuboidal epithelial cells are exactly located between the capillary and the ventricle. As all capillaries present within the brain, the capillaries of the choroid plexus have a wall formed by single cells responsible for ready transportation of ions and molecules to and from the choroid plexus capillary. Tight-gap junctions hold the choroid plexus epithelial cells together. These gap junctions prevent substances from entering or leaving the CSF; thus, the choroid plexus acts as a blood-CSF barrier. Lastly, although the CSF originates in the ventricles, this fluid flows through to the ventricles and then surrounds the brain and the spinal cord.

5. NPs for brain drug delivery

Over the last several years, researches have engineered a variety of NPs that can potentially deliver therapies and/or imaging agents directly into the brain [14, 42, 44–48]. It is really challenging to get these nanoparticles across the BBB to treat a CNS disease in sufficient amount and without causing major side effects on healthy brain cells. NPs are available in many sizes and shapes and they can have a positive, negative or neutral surface charge (**Figures 2, 3**). Their core can be made of a variety of materials such as biological, synthetic or energy receptive. NPs can also be coated with specialized molecules that allow them to interact with their environment. NPs can also be loaded with therapeutic molecules that are released in a controlled way and, at the same time, retain the drug stability and prevent them from degradation once in the blood. Therefore, for an efficient drug delivery into the CNS, it is very important to engineer NPs with the following properties: (i) small size (NP diameter should be smaller than 100 nm); (ii) biocompatible, biodegradable, nontoxic and noninflammatory; (iii) prolonged circulation time in the body; (iv) stable in the plasma; (v) protect the cargo such as small molecules, peptides [43, 49–51], proteins or nucleic acids from degradation; (vi) targetability to the BBB and (vii) controlled drug release [44].

One of the most important and challenging characteristics in engineering NPs is their functionalization. Active targeting of NPs can be achieved by attaching onto their surface, in a highly controlled way, specific molecules such as monoclonal antibody, RNA aptamers, transferrin, lactoferrin and peptides (**Figure 2**). An example of such active NP is the extensive

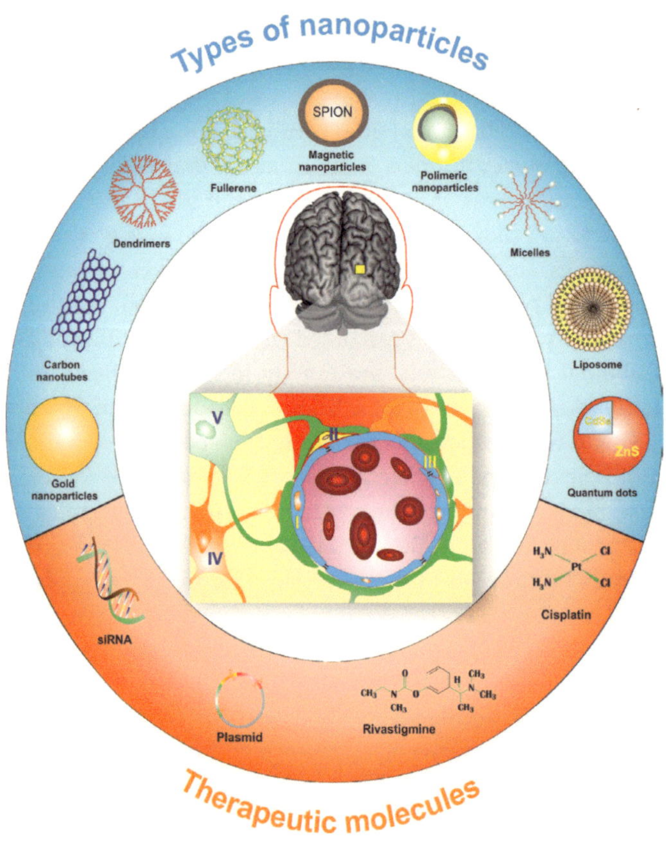

Figure 3. Types of nanoparticles for brain delivery. Enhancing brain drug delivery with the use of several nanocarriers, able to carry the most diverse kind of molecules.

use of cell penetrating peptides such as SynB vectors, Tat and penetratin that were successfully used to target the BBB [52–55]. In fact, a huge variety of molecules that increased targeting strategies to the BBB such as growth factors (e.g., vascular endothelial growth factor; epidermal growth factor) [56], albumin [57], insulin [58], lactoferrin [59], transferrin [60], angiopep-2 [61] and biotin-binding proteins has been reported [62]. Targetability is usually associated with nanoparticles with prolonged circulation time. This characteristic is achieved by coating the surface of NPs with hydrophilic polymers such a polyethylene glycol (PEG), poly(acryloylmorpholine), poly-N-vinylpyrrolidones, polyvinyl alcohol and poly[N-(2-hydroxypropyl) methacrylamide] [63] (**Figures 2, 3**). Among these polymers, PEG is still the most useful polymer in obtaining long circulating NP. The attachment of polymers onto the surface of NPs works by preventing NPs interaction with opsonins present at the plasma and, in this way, impeding their capture and subsequent clearance from the body. However, it was observed that the blood clearance phenomenon is accelerated after repetitive administration of clinically used PEGylated NPs due to the induction of production of antibodies (the NPs used in these studies were PEGylated liposomes) [64, 65]. Moreover, PEGylated NPs are particularly useful for neurological disease treatment, since the long-circulating NPs into the brain by diverse mechanisms were observed. Nevertheless, for brain tumors, reliance on the enhanced permeability and retention (EPR) effect for drug delivery strategies faces several challenges, since the accumulation of NPs at the tumor site is very low [66].

Due to their ability to carry hydrophilic, hydrophobic and/or lipophilic compounds and high specificity, the use of NPs provides a very efficient platform for drug delivery into the CNS. The most popular nanocarrier studied for brain drug delivery is liposomes and several liposomal formulations are clinically available or tested at different clinical trial phases [14]. Liposomes are spherical concentric vesicles, consisting of at least one lipid bilayer, enclosing an aqueous compartment. This nanocarrier has been employed for therapeutically active compounds delivery soon after its discovery by Bangham in the early 1960s. This NP has been successfully engineered for a variety of brain neurodegenerative disorders and brain tumors. For a detailed overview of liposome-based strategies to drug delivery across the BBB, we refer the reader to Vieira and Gamarra's article [14].

One of the breakthroughs of nanoparticles formulations is to target the nanocarriers to deliver their cargo into the brain. The brain endothelial cells contain several targets as discussed earlier that are explored on the studies of nanoparticles for brain delivery. Each of these targets could be specific for a brain disease or brain diseases. For example, transferrin has been described as the BBB-targeting ligand in studies of nanoparticle formulations [67, 68]. Transferrin is a glycoprotein (80 kDa) that binds to the transferrin receptor and is taken across the BBB via Receptor mediated endocytosis (RME). Indeed, these studies demonstrated that transferrin conjugated to liposomes exhibited a significant increase in the concentration of therapeutic molecules delivered by NPs into the brain when compared to the administration of the drug alone. In addition, broad ranges of nanocarriers with different shapes, sizes and surface properties have been developed for the transport of therapeutic or imaging molecules across the BBB. These also include carbon nanotubes [69, 70], micelles [71], dendrimers [72, 73], nanofibers [74, 75], polymer [46, 76], gold [77] and iron oxide nanoparticles [78] NPs (**Figure 3**).

Although nanotechnology-based strategies to get into the brain have shown progress in animal models, the translation of passive- and active-targeting delivery strategies into clinical studies is still questionable. This might be due to the random nature of receptor-ligand interactions and/or ineffective release of drug from the nanocarrier at the targeted site [79]. Therefore, the development of multifunctional nanoparticles is becoming possible due to the engineering of stimuli-responsive systems that are able to control the release of their cargo and drug distribution in response to specific stimuli such as magnetic field, light, changes in pH, variations in temperature, among others (**Figure 2**).

6. NPs in context of brain neurological diseases

Getting NPs into CNS is not an easy task. As discussed earlier, the BBB is the main structure responsible for brain protection and homeostasis. In addition, it is important to mention that in neurological diseases, several impairments of this structure occur, leading to the perpetuation of the inflammatory cycle that damages neuronal cells and neurodegeneration [80] Moreover, the BBB breakdown can occur, which is clearly a consequence of an ischemic stroke that occurred [81] due to an obstruction within a blood vessel that supplies the brain with oxygen and several nutrients, leading to brain cell death.

In other cases, especially in chronic neurological diseases such as Alzheimer's disease (AD) and Parkinson's disease (PD), it remains unclear how these diseases promote the BBB impairment [32]. Importantly, these modifications in the BBB structure should be taken into consideration when you are planning the engineering of effective multifunctional NPs for brain delivery. In this context, NPs have been designed to cross the BBB and this new technology has some applications so far in the treatment of Alzheimer's and Parkinson's diseases, stroke and brain tumors, which are discussed in the following section.

6.1. Stroke

Stroke is a serious disease that occurs when some or all of the blood supply to a part of the brain is restricted or cut off and, therefore, this can lead to disability, brain injury or death. Thus, the loss of oxygen and nutrients provided by the blood causing the loss of brain function is a stroke also known as cerebral ischemia. There are two ways to disturb the blood supply to the brain (**Figure 4**). The most common type occurs when there is a stoppage of blood flow to a part of the brain due to a blood clot. This cause of strokes accounts for 85% of all cases and it is known as ischemic stroke. The second cause of stroke, that is not as common as the ischemic stroke, but still very serious, happens when one of the blood vessels that is a part of the cerebral circulation supplying the brain ruptures. This kind of stroke is called a hemorrhagic stroke. In addition, "hemorrhagic" refers to a sudden torrential bleeding outburst. However, regardless of whether it is an ischemic stroke or a hemorrhagic stroke, the brain cells start to malfunction after some minutes due to the lack of oxygen and nutrients owing to improper blood flow or improper blood supply.

http://dx.doi.org/10.5772/intechopen.76922

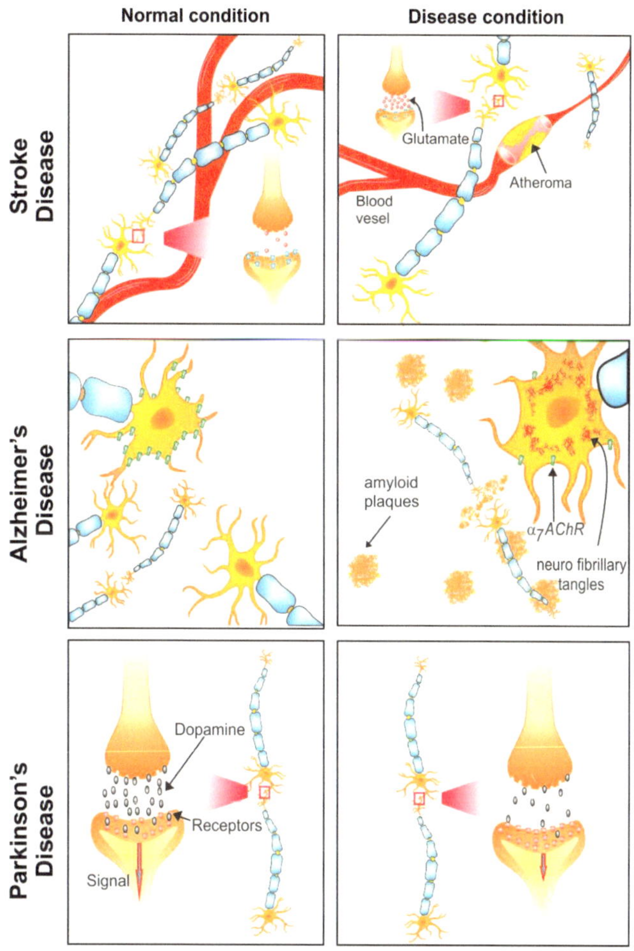

Figure 4. Schematic representation of the main event causing ischemic stroke, Alzheimer's and Parkinson's disease. (Adapted from Alvarim et al. [82]) ischemic stroke is caused by the interruption of the blood flow, depriving the brain of oxygen and some nutrients. For Alzheimer's disease, the main characteristic of this disease is the presence of neurofibrillary tangles and amyloid plaques in the brain, leading to shrinkage of some structures of the brain such as the hippocampus and the enlargement of the brain ventricles, resulting in neurodegeneration. In Parkinson's disease, substantia nigra dopamine neurons are lost.

There is also a related condition called the transient ischemic attack (TIA), also known as a mini-stroke. It is essentially a temporary interruption of blood flow to a part of the brain often lasting between 30 m and several hours. Therefore, the symptoms of TIA and stroke are similar. However, the difference is that a TIA does not actually destroy brain cells and it does not cause permanent disability. Nevertheless, it is often a warning signal that an individual is at risk of having a stroke in the near future. One of the key differences is that a TIA will resolve, whereas, if an individual has a stroke, he/she may not gain normal functioning again for weeks or months, or maybe even for the rest of his/her life.

Nevertheless, the cellular and molecular mechanisms of a stroke episode have been very well known due to the development of several experimental animal models of ischemic stroke [83]. From the studies with these animal models, it was observed that during ischemic stroke, first occurs the opening of the BBB for a short time period. Then, occurs a refractory interval, followed by a reopening of the BBB, but this time for a long period [84] The reopening of the BBB is the step responsible for the activation of the endothelium, leukocyte recruitment, reactive oxygen species (ROS) and cytokine productions and edema formation [85], leading to an inflammatory response and the BBB breakdown and cell death upon stroke [86]. Moreover, dysregulation of tight-junction proteins is also observed during ischemic stroke, due to their degradation by matrix metalloproteinases, which are involved in the process of BBB extracellular degradation, leading to an increase in the permeability of the brain structure [32].

Therefore, besides the BBB itself being an excellent target for itself for treating ischemic stroke, the design of effective drug delivery systems has also to take into consideration the cellular and molecular mechanisms described earlier. One of the strategies described in the literature to overcome neuronal tissue damage after a stroke event is the use of multifunctional NPs to deliver neuroprotective drugs into the brain, since the majority of neuroprotective drugs do not cross the BBB in their free form. For example, the inactive caspase-3 activation in the brain cells likely decreases the probability of brain cell damage after a stroke event. Although it was shown that some peptide inhibitors of caspase are effective compounds in promoting neuroprotection, they cannot readily cross the BBB. For this purpose, a positively charged NP of chitosan conjugated with transferrin receptor was designed to deliver the relatively specific caspase-3 inhibitor N-benzyloxycarbonyl-Asp(OMe)-Glu(OMe)-Val-Asp(OMe)-fluoromethyl ketone (Z-DEVD-FMK) across the BBB [36]. By clearly reducing the caspase 3-activity *in vivo*, this formulation was also readily transported across the BBB (less than 1 h) and it decreased neurological deficits and the infarcted area, proving to be a very promising formulation [27].

In the same way, several other compounds have been described to provide neuroprotection and to prevent neurodegeneration. One of these compounds is the Tanshinone IIA that has demonstrated neuroprotective effects against ischemic injury [87]. However, its use in the treatment of this disease is limited due to the compound's low solubility in aqueous medium, short-half circulation in the plasma and inability to cross the BBB. To overcome these limitations, Tanshinone IIA was successfully conjugated to PEGylated-cationic bovine serum albumin. These nanoparticles were able to cross the BBB *in vivo*, as a significant decreasing in the infarcted volume was observed. In addition, a reduction in the neutrophil infiltration and neuronal apoptosis was observed [88]. The authors also explored the molecular mechanisms by which this formulation conferred neuroprotection. It seems that the mechanism of action of this formulation in the brain is related to the down-regulation of pro-inflammatory cytokines (mainly IL-8 and TNF-α), to the up-regulation of anti-inflammatory cytokines (mainly transforming growth factor-β1 and IL-10) and to the reduction or inhibition of mRNA and proteins (mainly GFAP, MMP-9, COX-2, p38MAPK, ERK1/2 and JNK) [88].

As a last example, adenosine is also a powerful molecule that has demonstrated neuroprotection to the brain after an ischemic stroke event. This molecule also presents as limitations short-life time in the plasma and inability to cross the BBB. Here, adenosine was conjugated to the lipid-squalene and, then, yielded negatively charged NPs, showing promising results [89]. *In vivo* experiments showed that this formulation was able to extend adenosine circulation time in the plasma, interact with the neurovascular unit, enhance animal neurological deficit scores and decrease the size of the infarcted area [89].

6.2. Alzheimer's disease

It has been estimated that AD, only in the USA, affects over 5.5 million people. Moreover, Alzheimer's AD is the most common cause of dementia [90]. Dementia is a serious brain disease that has as major symptoms deterioration in memory, behavior and thinking. In 2015, dementia affected 47.5 million people worldwide. Most were over the age of 60. The United States data related to AD account that this disease was the sixth highest cause of death in 2005. It was also observed that 1 in 3 seniors who died had AD or other kinds of dementia. It is also expected that the number of people with Alzheimer's will grow as the population of those over the age of 65 rises. In 2015, Alzheimer's disease and other dementia cost the nation $226 billion and by 2050 this may rise to $1.1 trillion [90].

AD was named after the German physician Dr. Alois Alzheimer who presented a case history before an important medical meeting. In 1901, he was closely following a 51-year-old woman patient with a mental disorder, the manifestations of which were language problems and memory loss. After her death, Dr. Alzheimer took a serious examination of her brain and found the presence of plaques and tangles that today characterize AD [91]. This disease accounts for about 60–80% of the dementia cases. In most cases, Alzheimer's clinical manifestations first appear after the age of 65. However, Alzheimer's disease is not considered normal aging although the greatest risk factor of developing the disease is increased age. This is actually the greatest known risk factor for developing AD. However, as mentioned earlier, Alzheimer's is not a normal part of aging. It was observed that a greater proportion of patients over 85 years have AD compared to those over 65 years as AD is more likely to affect older individuals. Dominant genes that are transmitted through generations cause less than 5% of Alzheimer's. However, family risk is the second biggest factor for the development of AD after a certain age. In these families, individuals usually present symptoms of Alzheimer's before the age of 65 and these symptoms sometimes appear in their 30s. This form of AD that is hereditary and marked by Alzheimer's symptoms at an early age is called early-onset familial Alzheimer's disease (EOFAD). To date, mutations in presenilin (PS1 on chromosome 14 and PS2 on chromosome 1) and the amyloid precursor protein gene (APP) on chromosome 21 have been associated with EOFAD. All these three gene mutations (PS1/PS2/APP) affect the pathway in amyloid precursor protein synthesis, which leads to the increase of production of Aβ, creating plaques in the brain [92]. Additionally, there are certain genes such as apoE gene on chromosome 19 that increase the susceptibility to AD. There are three forms of the apoE gene: APOE2, APOE3 and APOE4, the last one being the one associated with a high risk for developing AD. Actually, an individual with two copies of this gene is at three to eight more risk than people with one copy of this gene.

The human brain contains about 100 billion neurons that communicate to one another via synapses, when a burst of chemicals called neurotransmitters are released [93]. The neurotransmitters are synthesized into the synaptic gap. Then, neurotransmitters move across these synaptic gaps between neurons and bind to receptor sites on the dendrites of the next neuron. Unfortunately, neurons are the type of cells affected by AD. To date, scientists still do not know exactly the causes of AD and how this process begins. However, according to recent studies, it appears to be likely that astrocytes' activation contributes to the neuroinflammatory component responsible for the damage of neurons decades before the issue becomes obvious [94].

Abnormal structures called β-amyloid plaques and neurofibrillary tangles are classical biological hallmarks of the disease [91]. The formation of extracellular β-amyloid plaques occurs when amyloid precursor protein in the neuron cell membrane is cleaved at different positions, releasing small fragments called amyloid β (Aβ) that are highly toxic to the neurons and also interfere with the function of the brain cells [95]. Neurofibrillary tangles, on the other hand, are aggregates of hyperphosphorylate of a microtubule-associated protein known as tau. Tau protein, which in normal cells is responsible for helping nerve cells transport nutrients and maintain their proper shape, is altered in AD and, as a consequence, the transport of nutrients and other essential supplies into the neuron is affected, causing its death. At the same time, the health neurons start working less effectively. After some time, these neurons start losing their capacity to function and communicate to one another and, eventually, they die. Then, the harm may spread to structures in the brain such as hippocampus and entorhinal cortex, which are crucial areas of the brain responsible for forming new memories, thus causing memory loss. As neurons continue to die, affected areas of the brain begin to shrinks and brain functions are lost (**Figure 4**).

The BBB impairment in AD has been controversial [96]. However, several studies carried out in AD patients or AD animal models have been suggesting that the cause of cerebrovascular alterations in the BBB of the diseased brains is the accumulation of Aβ peptide [97–99]. Nevertheless, there are also studies suggesting that the BBB impairment is the cause of neurodegeneration, since the dysfunction of the brain structure in AD animal models was observed before Aβ aggregates were accumulated [100]. In any case, both hypotheses for the dysfunction of the BBB consider as a secondary event the tauopathies. However, a study reported that the tau filaments alone are able to start the disruption of the BBB and when it was deregulated, the BBB integrity was recovered [101].

Currently, there are no drug treatments that can cure AD. For this reason, approaches for treating AD are focused more on therapeutic interventions that alleviate symptoms, slow down or delay the progression of the disease, improving the patient's quality of life. To date, there are two types of medications for Alzheimer's treatment: acetylcholinesterase inhibitors (Aricept, Reminyl, Exelon and Cognex) and N-Methyl-D-aspartate (NMDA) receptor antagonist (Namenda). Nevertheless, the administration of these therapeutic molecules is associated with severe side effects. Thus, it would be desirable to develop drugs that can efficiently deliver these drugs into the brain. Moreover, there are also several studies showing that neuroprotective peptides might be an excellent compound for AD therapy, since they have shown to be able to break down and degrade Aβ plaques.

Multifunctional NPs are a good option to carry these peptides, since nanocarriers can protect them from degrading into the plasma by proteolytic enzymes and increase their stability in the serum. For example, PEG-PLA NPs were able to protect the neuroprotective peptide NAPVSIPQ from degradation. However, just NPs modified with B6 peptide (similar to transferrin) were able to cross the blood-brain barrier in mice and successfully deliver the neuroprotective peptide into the brain [102]. Moreover, it was observed that the treatment with this formulation improved cholinergic function and ameliorated spatial learning of AD mouse model [102]. In the same way, the nerve growth factor (NGF) has also been explored as a good drug for treating AD, although it is not able to cross the BBB. For this purpose, NGF was encapsulated into PBCA NPs, decorated with polysorbate 80 [103]. These NPs presented very promising results, since they were able to reach the mice brain parenchyma in less than 1 h after administration and these nanocarriers also proved to be able to improve recognition and memory of mice and to reduce by almost 40% the PD symptoms such as rigidity, tremor and oligokinesia in animal models [103]. Coenzyme Q10, a powerful antioxidant macromolecule, has also been explored at AD therapy. In this way, this coenzyme was encapsulated within PLGA NPs decorated with trimethylates chitosan. The results showed that these nanoparticles were able to cross the BBB and accumulate in the choroid plexus, ventricles and cortex. Moreover, the authors also observed an improvement in the cognitive and spatial memory performance of AD mice models and a significant reduction of senile plaques and levels of ROS [104].

6.3. Parkinson's disease

After Alzheimer's, PD is the second most common disease in terms of neurodegenerative diseases. As the aging population increases, the number of people with this disease is expected to rise. It affects 0.3% and 1% of the population worldwide over the age of 40 years and 65 years, respectively. Pathologically, PD is characterized by progressive loss of muscle control, which leads to tremor of hands, bradykinesia, rigidity and postural instability [105] Motor impairment in PD can also cause hypomimia, which is the decreased degree of facial expression. Dysphagia and hypophonia, which are disruption of the swallowing process and lack of coordination in the vocal musculature, are also common features in PD. Other symptoms also include ophthalmologic complaints such as blurred vision and gate. It is important to mention that all these signs and symptoms are a result of affected areas that occur within the brain, especially in an area known as basal ganglia [105].

Thus, PD is a result of problems that occur within the basal ganglia. The basal ganglia is a collection of nuclei located deep beneath the cerebral cortex and it is responsible for the correct execution of voluntary muscle movements and learned movement patterns. The components of basal ganglia are caudate nucleus and putamen (dorsal striatum); nucleus accumbens and olfactory tubercule (ventral striatum), ventral pallidum, globus pallidus, subthalamic nucleus and substantia nigra. In PD, the basal ganglia is disrupted, causing degeneration of dopaminergic neurons located at the substantia nigra. Essentially, it is considered a disease of the basal ganglia because what happens is that when the cerebral cortex wants to initiate a movement, the basal ganglia receives these signals and sends it back the motor cortex via the thalamus. Through various pathways, the substantia nigra is connected with nuclei in basal ganglia. The basal ganglia plays an essential role in integrating multiple input signals to modulate the output of the motor cortex. Inhibitory or excitatory connections can occur in this process. Thus, the loss of dopamine from substantia nigra in this process underlies the symptoms described earlier [105].

At the beginning, researches believed that the BBB did not suffer any kind of alteration during the disease development [106]. Surprisingly, tracking compounds such as [^{11}C]-verapamil and benserazide in the brain of PD patients or PD animal models, it was observed that the concentration of these compounds in the brain was increased, what does not happen in the brain of health patients or animals since these drugs are not able to cross the BBB [107]. In addition to this, a good correlation between the albumin ratio and progressive BB integrity loss in the brain of patients with PD was observed [107]. Moreover, other signals of the BBB impairment such as vascular alterations and blood flow deficiencies were reported [108]. Most important, the increased expression of vascular endothelial growth factor (VEGF) was directly correlated with the high amount of blood vessels presented in the damaged dopaminergic neurons in the brain of monkeys [109]. Later, it was observed that the injection of VEGF into the substantia nigra in the brain of rats disrupted the BBB, leading to a strong inflammation response and loss of dopaminergic neurons [110]. Lastly, alpha-synuclein aggregates are the central hallmark of PD and their accumulation seems to be correlated with the downregulation of the P-glycoprotein (**Figure 4**) [111]. Moreover, higher concentration of some metals like iron was found in the brain of PD patients and PD animal models because of the higher levels of lactoferrin receptor in the substantia nigra dopaminergic neurons of the diseased brain [32].

Currently, there is no cure for PD. However, there are drugs that work to decrease and relieve the symptoms of PD and maintain the quality of life of the patient. The most effective treatment for PD is the use of the drug levodopa—also called L-dopa—or dopamine that is both able to restore or increase the concentration of dopamine in the basal ganglia. But here, we want to discuss an article that explored the increased expression of lactoferrin in some region of the brain in PD patients [112]. In this way, a PAMAM and PEG NPs were developed, coated with lactoferrin to the delivery of a plasmid of human glial cell line-derived neurotrophic factor plasmid (GDNF), since GDNF is a promising factor in treating PD, but as all plasmids are unable to cross the BBB. These multifunctional nanoparticles were able to not only cross the brain barrier but also effectively deliver the plasmid into the brain, since a neuroprotective effect on dopaminergic neurons and improvement of locomotor activities in AD animal models was observed [113]. Another example is the encapsulation of urocortin (hormone-related peptide) in PEGylated-PLGA NPs covered by lactoferrin. From the results presented, this formulation was able to quickly cross the BBB and to promote protection to the dopaminergic neurons and improve locomotor functional deficits [114].

7. Conclusions

Nanotechnology in the field of medicine has brought a variety of new ways to treat and/or detect diseases [13, 115, 116]. Currently, engineered pharmaceutical NPs demonstrated abilities such as long blood circulation time in the body fluids for their accumulation at disease sites with leaky vasculature [117]; specific targeted drug delivery to the pathological area due to the surface functionalization of NPs with ligands such as antibodies [118]; contrast properties due to their unique capacity of carrying contrast agents allowing their tracking *in vivo* [119]; drug delivery from the particles responsive to a specific stimuli [79] and others. The tremendous advances in nanomedicine during the past decade have significantly advanced on the engineering of nanoparticles that combine several of these characteristics, known as multifunctional NPs. Long-circulating and target-specific NPs capable of prolonged circulation time in the blood and targeted delivery of drug to the brain and *in vivo* imaging represent one example of a multifunctional nanocarrier [44].

Moreover, we hope this chapter was a bridge between nanotechnology and central nervous systems disorders, since multifunctional NPs have a great potential in the treatment of neurological disorders in the near future [14, 44, 120]. However, as discussed, the BBB is one of the major obstacles to the delivery of drugs into the brain and, consequently, for the treatment of neurological diseases [48, 121]. The BBB is composed of very tightly connected endothelial cells and a variety of transporters [15, 17, 120, 122]. This results in a highly selective permeability barrier that separates the circulating blood from the cerebral parenchyma, thus limiting the entry of drugs into the brain. As discussed earlier, several multifunctional NPs for delivering therapeutic and/or imaging molecules into the brain have been developed [44, 47, 123]. Thus, this part of the chapter was organized in a way to carry the reader through the fundamentals of common neurological diseases such as Alzheimer's, Parkinson's and cerebral ischemia and their potential treatments with these kinds of NPs [44, 68, 88, 102, 124–139]. The purpose was to analyze some of the major scientific data indexed in PubMed, Web of Science and Scopus to explore different approaches engineered to transport and deliver imaging or therapeutic molecules to the brain by using multifunctional NPs technology. In this way, our gathered data on different strategies for the delivery of drugs across the BBB using multifunctional NPs were reviewed, discussed and grouped in self-explanatory figures. Results of our analysis from some research articles on our search showed that several strategies have been used to deliver several therapeutic compounds to the brain by these NPs. Functionalization of the surface of these NPs by covalent ligation of macromolecules such as antibodies, RNA aptamers as well peptides is an effective method for receptor targeting nanocarriers, which allows their BBB-penetration and the efficient delivery of their cargo specifically to the disease site. Additionally, methods for the development of multifunctional NPs that can respond to external stimuli were employed, concluding that the development of multifunctional NPs for treating neurological disorders still is at its infancy, although these systems have a huge chance to revolutionize the ways that brain diseases are treated.

Author details

Débora Braga Vieira and Lionel Fernel Gamarra*

*Address all correspondence to: lionelgamarra7@gmail.com

Hospital Israelita Albert Einstein, São Paulo, Brazil

References

[1] Kendall M, Lynch I. Long-term monitoring for nanomedicine implants and drugs. Nature Nanotechnology. 2016;**11**(3):206-210. Available at: http://www.nature.com/doifinder/10.1038/nnano.2015.341

[2] Lee D-E et al. Multifunctional nanoparticles for multimodal imaging and theragnosis. Chemical Society Reviews. 2012;**41**(7):2656-2672. Available at: http://xlink.rsc.org/?DOI=C2CS15261D

[3] Chapman S et al. Nanoparticles for cancer imaging: The good, the bad, and the promise. Nano Today. 2013;**8**(5):454-460. Available at: http://dx.doi.org/10.1016/j.nantod.2013.06.001

[4] Chen ZG. Small-molecule delivery by nanoparticles for anticancer therapy. Trends in Molecular Medicine. 2010;**16**(12):594-602. Available at: http://dx.doi.org/10.1016/j.molmed.2010.08.001

[5] Mudshinge SR et al. Nanoparticles: Emerging carriers for drug delivery. Saudi Pharmaceutical Journal. 2011;**19**(3):129-141. Available at: http://dx.doi.org/10.1016/j.jsps.2011.04.001

[6] Vieira DB, Gamarra LF. Advances in the use of nanocarriers for cancer diagnosis and treatment. Einstein (São Paulo). 2016a;**14**(1):99-103. Available at: http://www.scielo.br/scielo.php?script=sci_arttext&pid=S1679-45082016000100099&lng=en&nrm=iso&tlng=en

[7] Wagner V et al. The emerging nanomedicine landscape. Nature Biotechnology. 2006;**24**(10):1211-1217. Available at: http://www.nature.com/doifinder/10.1038/nbt1006-1211 [Accessed May 11, 2016]

[8] Petros RA, DeSimone JM. Strategies in the design of nanoparticles for therapeutic applications. Nature Reviews Drug Discovery. 2010;**9**(8):615-627. Available at: http://www.nature.com/doifinder/10.1038/nrd2591 [Accessed May 12, 2016]

[9] Peer D et al. Nanocarriers as an emerging platform for cancer therapy. Nature Nanotechnology. 2007;**2**(12):751-760. Available at: http://www.nature.com/doifinder/10.1038/nnano.2007.387 [Accessed May 13, 2016]

[10] Schöttler S et al. Protein adsorption is required for stealth effect of poly(ethylene glycol)- and poly(phosphoester)-coated nanocarriers. Nature Nanotechnology. 2016;**11**(4):372-377. Available at: http://www.nature.com/doifinder/10.1038/nnano.2015.330 [Accessed May 13, 2016]

[11] Butcher NJ, Mortimer GM, Minchin RF. Drug delivery: Unravelling the stealth effect. Nature Nanotechnology. 2016;**11**(4):310-311. Available at: http://www.nature.com/doifinder/10.1038/nnano.2016.6 [Accessed May 13, 2016]

[12] Steichen SD, Caldorera-Moore M, Peppas NA. A review of current nanoparticle and targeting moieties for the delivery of cancer therapeutics. European Journal of Pharmaceutical Sciences. 2013;**48**(3):416-427. Available at: http://linkinghub.elsevier.com/retrieve/pii/S0928098712004782 [Accessed May 13, 2016]

[13] Torchilin VP. Multifunctional, stimuli-sensitive nanoparticulate systems for drug delivery. Nature Reviews. Drug Discovery. 2014;**13**(11):813-827. Available at: http://www.ncbi.nlm.nih.gov/pubmed/25287120

[14] Vieira DB, Gamarra LF. Getting into the brain: Liposome-based strategies for effective drug delivery across the blood–brain barrier. International Journal of Nano-medicine. 2016b;**11**:5381-5414. Available at: https://www.dovepress.com/getting-into-the-brain-liposome-based-strategies-for-effective-drug-de-peer-reviewed-article-IJN [Accessed October 24, 2016]

[15] Ballabh P, Braun A, Nedergaard M. The blood-brain barrier: An overview: Structure, regulation, and clinical implications. Neurobiology of Disease. 2004;**16**(1):1-13

[16] Hawkins BT. The blood-brain barrier/neurovascular unit in health and disease. Pharmacological Reviews. 2005;**57**(2):173-185. Available at: http://pharmrev.aspetjournals.org/cgi/doi/10.1124/pr.57.2.4

[17] Abbott NJ et al. Structure and function of the blood-brain barrier. Neurobiology of Disease. 2010;**37**(1):13-25. Available at: http://dx.doi.org/10.1016/j.nbd.2009.07.030

[18] Perea G, Sur M, Araque A. Neuron-glia networks: Integral gear of brain function. Frontiers in Cellular Neuroscience. 2014;**8**:378. Available at: http://www.ncbi.nlm.nih.gov/pubmed/25414643 [Accessed September 19, 2016]

[19] Kimelberg HK, Nedergaard M. Functions of astrocytes and their potential as therapeutic targets. Neurotherapeutics. 2010;**7**(4):338-353. Available at: http://www.ncbi.nlm.nih.gov/pubmed/20880499 [Accessed September 13, 2016]

[20] Armulik A et al. Pericytes regulate the blood–brain barrier. Nature. 2010;**468**(7323):557-561. Available at: http://www.ncbi.nlm.nih.gov/pubmed/20944627 [Accessed September 20, 2016]

[21] Lau LW et al. Pathophysiology of the brain extracellular matrix: A new target for remyelination. Nature Reviews Neuroscience. 2013;**14**(10):722-729. Available at: http://www.ncbi.nlm.nih.gov/pubmed/23985834 [Accessed September 20, 2016]

[22] Pardridge WM. Blood–brain barrier delivery. Drug Discovery Today. 2007;**12**(1-2):54-61. Available at: http://linkinghub.elsevier.com/retrieve/pii/S1359644606004363

[23] Pandey PK, Sharma AK, Gupta U. Blood brain barrier: An overview on strategies in drug delivery, realistic in vitro modeling and in vivo live tracking. Tissue Barriers. 2016;**4**(1):e1129476. Available at: http://www.tandfonline.com/doi/full/10.1080/21688370.2015.1129476 [Accessed October 25, 2016]

[24] Decuzzi P et al. Size and shape effects in the biodistribution of intravascularly injected particles. Journal of Controlled Release. 2010;**141**(3):320-327. Available at: http://linkinghub.elsevier.com/retrieve/pii/S0168365909007093 [Accessed October 26, 2016]

[25] Gao X et al. Overcoming the blood–brain barrier for delivering drugs into the brain by using adenosine receptor Nanoagonist. ACS Nano. 2014;**8**(4):3678-3689. Available at: http://pubs.acs.org/doi/abs/10.1021/nn5003375 [Accessed October 26, 2016]

[26] Guerrero S et al. Improving the brain delivery of gold nanoparticles by conjugation with an amphipathic peptide. Nanomedicine. 2010;**5**(6):897-913. Available at: http://www.futuremedicine.com/doi/abs/10.2217/nnm.10.74 [Accessed October 26, 2016]

[27] Karatas H et al. A Nanomedicine transports a peptide Caspase-3 inhibitor across the blood-brain barrier and provides Neuroprotection. Journal of Neuroscience. 2009;**29**(44):13761-13769. Available at: http://www.jneurosci.org/cgi/doi/10.1523/JNEUROSCI.4246-09.2009 [Accessed October 26, 2016]

[28] Reimold I et al. Delivery of nanoparticles to the brain detected by fluorescence microscopy. European Journal of Pharmaceutics and Biopharmaceutics. 2008;**70**(2):627-632. Available at: http://linkinghub.elsevier.com/retrieve/pii/S093964110800180X [Accessed October 26, 2016]

[29] Shilo M et al. Transport of nanoparticles through the blood–brain barrier for imaging and therapeutic applications. Nanoscale. 2014;**6**(4):2146-2152. Available at: http://xlink.rsc.org/?DOI=C3NR04878K [Accessed October 26, 2016]

[30] Bramini M et al. Imaging approach to mechanistic study of nanoparticle interactions with the blood–brain barrier. ACS Nano. 2014;**8**(5):4304-4312. Available at: http://pubs.acs.org/doi/abs/10.1021/nn5018523 [Accessed October 26, 2016]

[31] Georgieva JV et al. Surface characteristics of nanoparticles determine their intracellular fate in and processing by human blood–brain barrier endothelial cells in vitro. Molecular Therapy. 2011;**19**(2):318-325. Available at: http://www.nature.com/doifinder/10.1038/mt.2010.236 [Accessed October 26, 2016]

[32] Saraiva C et al. Nanoparticle-mediated brain drug delivery: Overcoming blood–brain barrier to treat neurodegenerative diseases. Journal of Controlled Release. 2016;**235**:34-47. Available at: http://linkinghub.elsevier.com/retrieve/pii/S0168365916303236 [Accessed October 25, 2016]

[33] Cho H et al. Three-dimensional blood-brain barrier model for in vitro studies of Neurovascular Pathology. Scientific Reports. 2015;**5**:15222. Available at: http://www.nature.com/articles/srep15222 [Accessed October 26, 2016]

[34] Czupalla CJ, Liebner S, Devraj K. In vitro models of the blood-brain barrier. Methods in Molecular Biology (Clifton, N.J.). 2014;**1135**:415-437. Available at: http://www.ncbi.nlm.nih.gov/pubmed/24510883 [Accessed October 26, 2016]

[35] Liu Q et al. P-glycoprotein mediated efflux limits the transport of the novel anti-Parkinson's disease candidate drug FLZ across the physiological and PD pathological in vitro BBB models M. Ahmad, ed. PLoS One. 2014;**9**(7):e102442. Available at: http://dx.plos.org/10.1371/journal.pone.0102442 [Accessed October 26, 2016]

[36] Mendes B et al. Influence of glioma cells on a new co-culture in vitro blood–brain barrier model for characterization and validation of permeability. International Journal of Pharmaceutics. 2015;**490**(1-2):94-101. Available at: http://www.ncbi.nlm.nih.gov/pubmed/25981617 [Accessed October 26, 2016]

[37] Vogelgesang S, Jedlitschky G. In vitro models of the human blood-brain barrier and the impact of efflux transporters on neurological disorders: The work of Cioni et al. (2012). Frontiers in Psychiatry. 2014;**5**:128. Available at: http://www.ncbi.nlm.nih.gov/pubmed/25278908 [Accessed October 26, 2016]

[38] Aday S et al. Stem cell-based human blood–brain barrier models for drug discovery and delivery. Trends in Biotechnology. 2016;**34**(5):382-393. Available at: http://linkinghub.elsevier.com/retrieve/pii/S0167779916000044 [Accessed October 26, 2016]

[39] Cecchelli R et al. A stable and reproducible human blood-brain barrier model derived from hematopoietic stem cells R. Klein, ed. PLoS One. 2014;**9**(6):e99733. Available at: http://dx.plos.org/10.1371/journal.pone.0099733 [Accessed October 26, 2016]

[40] Gudmundsson OS, Nimkar K, Gangwar S, Siahaan T, Borchardt RT. Phenylpropionic acid-based cyclic prodrugs of opioid peptides that exhibit metabolic stability to peptidases and excellent cellular permeation. Pharmaceutical Research. 1999;**16**(1):16-23. Retrieved from http://www.ncbi.nlm.nih.gov/pubmed/9950273

[41] On NH, Kiptoo P, Siahaan TJ, Miller DW. Modulation of blood-brain barrier permeability in mice using synthetic E-cadherin peptide. Molecular Pharmaceutics. 2014. DOI: https://doi.org/10.1021/mp400624v

[42] Pavan B et al. Progress in drug delivery to the central nervous system by the prodrug approach. Molecules. 2008;**13**(5):1035-1065

[43] Soltero R. Oral protein and peptide drug delivery. In: Wang B, Siahaan TJ, Soltero R, editors. Drug Delivery Principles and Applications. NJ, USA: John Wiley & Sons, Inc; 2005. pp. 189-200

[44] Bhaskar S et al. Multifunctional Nanocarriers for diagnostics, drug delivery and targeted treatment across blood-brain barrier: Perspectives on tracking and neuroimaging. Particle and Fibre Toxicology. 2010;**7**:3

[45] Hu L. Prodrug approaches to drug delivery. In: Wang B, Siahaan TJ, Soltero R, editors. Drug Delivery: Principles and Application. New York: John Wiley & Sons, Inc; 2005. pp. 125-165

[46] Kreuter J. Drug delivery to the central nervous system by polymeric nanoparticles: What do we know? Advanced Drug Delivery Reviews. 2014;**71**(2013):2-14. Available at: http://dx.doi.org/10.1016/j.addr.2013.08.008

[47] Lai F, Fadda AM, Sinico C. Liposomes for brain delivery. Expert Opinion on Drug Delivery. 2013;**10**(7):1003-1022. Available at: http://www.pubmedcentral.nih.gov/articlerender.fcgi?artid=3588019&tool=pmcentrez&rendertype=abstract%5Cnhttp://www.ncbi.nlm.nih.gov/pubmed/24524555

[48] Stenehjem DD et al. Novel and emerging strategies in drug delivery for overcoming the blood-brain barrier. Future Medicinal Chemistry. 2009;**1**(9):1623-1641

[49] Iskandarsyah, Tejo BA, Tambunan USF, Verkhivker G, Siahaan TJ. Structural modifications of ICAM-1 cyclic peptides to improve the activity to inhibit heterotypic adhsion of T cells. Chemical Biology & Drug Design. 2008;**72**(1):27-33. DOI: 10.1111/j.1747-0285.2008.00676.x

[50] Prasasty VD, Tambunan USF, Siahaan TJ. Homology modeling and molecular dynam icsstudies of EC1 domain of VE-cadherin to elucidate docking interaction with cad-herin-derived peptide. OnLine Journal of Biological Sciences. 2014;**14**(2):155. DOI: 10.3844/ojbsci.2014.155.162

[51] Siahaan TJ. Increasing paracellular porosity by E-cadherin peptides: Discovery of bulge and groove regions in the EC1-domain of E-cadherin. Pharmaceutical Research. 2002;**19**(8):1170-1179. Retrieved from http://www.ncbi.nlm.nih.gov/pubmed/12240943

[52] Berry C. Intracellular delivery of nanoparticles via the HIV-1 tat peptide. Nanomedicine. 2008;**3**(3):357-365. Available at: http://www.ncbi.nlm.nih.gov/pubmed/18510430 [Accessed January 19, 2017]

[53] de la Fuente JM, Berry CC. Tat peptide as an efficient molecule to translocate gold nanoparticles into the cell nucleus. Bioconjugate Chemistry. 2005;**16**(5):1176-1180. Available at: http://www.ncbi.nlm.nih.gov/pubmed/16173795 [Accessed January 19, 2017]

[54] Mortensen LJ et al. In Vivo skin penetration of quantum dot nanoparticles in the murine model: The effect of UVR. Nano Letters. 2008;**8**(9):2779-2787. Available at: http://www.ncbi.nlm.nih.gov/pubmed/18687009 [Accessed January 19, 2017]

[55] Rao KS et al. TAT-conjugated nanoparticles for the CNS delivery of anti-HIV drugs. Biomaterials. 2008;**29**(33):4429-4438. Available at: http://www.ncbi.nlm.nih.gov/pubmed/18760470 [Accessed January 19, 2017]

[56] Ikeda E et al. Brain-specific expression of vascular endothelial growth factor 146 correlates with the blood-brain barrier induction in quail embryos. Developmental Neuroscience. 2008;**30**(5):331-339. Available at: http://www.ncbi.nlm.nih.gov/pubmed/18594132 [Accessed January 19, 2017]

[57] Lu W et al. Cationic albumin conjugated pegylated nanoparticle with its transcytosis ability and little toxicity against blood–brain barrier. International Journal of Pharmaceutics. 2005;**295**(1-2):247-260. Available at: http://www.ncbi.nlm.nih.gov/pubmed/15848009 [Accessed January 19, 2017]

[58] Witt KA et al. Insulin enhancement of opioid peptide transport across the blood-brain barrier and assessment of analgesic effect. The Journal of Pharmacology and Exper imental Therapeutics. 2000;**295**(3):972-978. Available at: http://www.ncbi.nlm.nih.gov/pubmed/11082431 [Accessed January 19, 2017]

[59] Hu K, Li J, Shen Y, Lu W, Gao X, Zhang Q, Jiang X. Lactoferrin-conjugated PEG-PLA nanoparticles with improved brain delivery: In vitro and in vivo evaluations. The Journal Control Release. 20 Feb 2009;**134**(1):55-61. DOI: 10.1016/j.jconrel.2008.10.016. Epub 2008 Nov 12. PubMed. PMID: 19038299

[60] Ulbrich K et al. Transferrin- and transferrin-receptor-antibody-modified nanoparticles enable drug delivery across the blood–brain barrier (BBB). European Journal of Pharmaceutics and Biopharmaceutics. 2009;**71**(2):251-256. Available at: http://www.ncbi.nlm.nih.gov/pubmed/18805484 [Accessed January 19, 2017]

[61] Demeule M et al. Involvement of the low-density lipoprotein receptor-related protein in the transcytosis of the brain delivery vector Angiopep-2. Journal of Neurochemistry. 2008;**106**(4):1534-1544. Available at: http://www.ncbi.nlm.nih.gov/pubmed/18489712 [Accessed January 19, 2017]

[62] Townsend SA et al. Tetanus toxin C fragment-conjugated nanoparticles for targeted drug delivery to neurons. Biomaterials. 2007;**28**(34):5176-5184. Available at: http://www.ncbi.nlm.nih.gov/pubmed/17854886 [Accessed January 19, 2017]

[63] Torchilin VP. Recent advances with liposomes as pharmaceutical carriers. Nature Reviews Drug Discovery. 2005;**4**(2):145-160. Available at: http://www.nature.com/doifinder/10.1038/nrd1632

[64] Ishida T, Atobe K, et al. Accelerated blood clearance of PEGylated liposomes upon repeated injections: Effect of doxorubicin-encapsulation and high-dose first injection. Journal of Controlled Release: Official Journal of the Controlled Release Society. 2006a;**115**(3):251-258. Available at: http://www.ncbi.nlm.nih.gov/pubmed/17045355 [Accessed January 23, 2017]

[65] Ishida T, Ichihara M, et al. Injection of PEGylated liposomes in rats elicits PEG-specific IgM, which is responsible for rapid elimination of a second dose of PEGylated liposomes. Journal of Controlled Release. 2006b;**112**(1):15-25. Available at: http://www.ncbi.nlm.nih.gov/pubmed/16515818 [Accessed January 19, 2017]

[66] Schwartzbaum JA et al. Epidemiology and molecular pathology of glioma. Nature Clinical Practice Neurology. 2006;**2**(9):494-503. Available at: http://www.nature.com/doifinder/10.1038/ncpneuro0289

[67] Chen Z-L et al. Transferrin-modified liposome promotes α-mangostin to penetrate the blood-brain barrier. Nanomedicine: Nanotechnology, Biology and Medi-cine. 2016; **12**(2):421-430. Available at: http://www.nanomedjournal.com/article/S15-49963415005936/fulltext [Accessed May 31, 2016]

[68] Zhao H et al. Postacute ischemia vascular endothelial growth factor transfer by transferrin-targeted liposomes attenuates ischemic brain injury after experimental stroke in rats. Human Gene Therapy. 2011;**22**(2):207-215. Available at: http://www.liebertonline.com/doi/abs/10.1089/hum.2010.111

[69] Al-Jamal KT et al. Functional motor recovery from brain ischemic insult by carbon nanotube-mediated siRNA silencing. Proceedings of the National Academy of Sciences of the United States of America. 2011;**108**(27):10952-10957

[70] Ren J et al. The targeted delivery of anticancer drugs to brain glioma by PEGylated oxidized multi-walled carbon nanotubes modified with angiopep-2. Biomaterials. 2012; **33**(11):3324-3333. Available at: http://dx.doi.org/10.1016/j.biomaterials.2012.01.025

[71] Morshed RA et al. The potential of polymeric micelles in the context of glioblastoma therapy. Frontiers in Pharmacology. 2013;**4 DEC**(December):1-15

[72] Perez-Martinez FC et al. Dendrimers as vectors for genetic material delivery to the nervous system. Current Medicinal Chemistry. 2012;**19**(29):5101-5108. Available at: http://www.eurekaselect.com/103736/article [Accessed September 17, 2015]

[73] Somani S, Dufès C. Applications of dendrimers for brain delivery and cancer therapy. Nanomedicine. 2014;**9**(15):2403-2414. Available at: http://www.futuremedicine.com/doi/abs/10.2217/nnm.14.130

[74] Tseng Y et al. Biodegradable drug-eluting poly[lactic- co -glycol acid] nanofibers for the sustainable delivery of vancomycin to brain tissue: In vitro and in vivo studies. ACS Chemical Neuroscience. 2013;**4**(9):1314-1321. Available at: http://pubs.acs.org/doi/abs/10.1021/cn400108q

[75] Xie J, Wang C-H. Electrospun micro- and nanofibers for sustained delivery of paclitaxel to treat C6 Glioma in vitro. Pharmaceutical Research. 2006;**23**(8):1817-1826. Available at: http://link.springer.com/10.1007/s11095-006-9036-z

[76] Patel T et al. Polymeric nanoparticles for drug delivery to the central nervous system. Advanced Drug Delivery Reviews. 2012;**64**(7):701-705. Available at: http://dx.doi.org/10.1016/j.addr.2011.12.006

[77] Li W, Chen X. Gold nanoparticles for photoacoustic imaging. Nanomedicine. 2015;**10**(2): 299-320. Available at: http://www.futuremedicine.com/doi/abs/10.2217/nnm.14.169

[78] Sharma HS et al. The role of functionalized magnetic Iron oxide nanoparticles in the central nervous system injury and repair: New potentials for Neuroprotection with Cerebrolysin therapy. Journal of Nanoscience and Nanotechnology. 2014;**14**(1):577-595. Available at: http://openurl.ingenta.com/content/xref?genre=article&issn=1533-4880&volume=14&issue=1&spage=577

[79] Mura S, Nicolas J, Couvreur P. Stimuli-responsive nanocarriers for drug delivery. Nature Materials. 2013;**12**(11):991-1003. Available at: http://dx.doi.org/10.1038/nmat3776

[80] Obermeier B, Daneman R, Ransohoff R. Development, maintenance and disruption of the blood-brain barrier. Nature Medicine. 2013;**19**:1584-1596

[81] Khatri R, McKinney AM, Swenson B, Janardhan V. Blood-brain barrier, reperfusion injury, and hemorrhagic transformation in acute ischemic stroke. Neurology. 2012;**79** (13 Suppl 1):S52-S57 Review

[82] Alvarim LT, Nucci LP, Mamani JB, Marti LC, Aguiar MF, Silva HR, Silva GS, Nucci-da-Silva MP, DelBel EA, Gamarra LF. Therapeutics with SPION-labeled stem cells for the main diseases related to brain aging: A systematic review. International Journal of Nanomedicine. 2014;**9**:3749-3770. DOI: 10.2147/IJN.S65616

[83] Sommer CJ. Ischemic stroke: Experimental models and reality. Acta Neuropathologica. 2017;**133**(2):245-261. DOI: 10.1007/s00401-017-1667-0

[84] Jiao H, Wang Z, Liu Y, Wang P, Xue Y. Specific role of tight junction proteins claudin-5, occludin, and ZO-1 of the blood-brain barrier in a focal cerebral ischemic insult. Journal of Molecular Neuroscience. 2011;**44**(2):130-139. DOI: 10.1007/s12031-011-9496-4

[85] Merali Z, Huang K, Mikulis D, Silver F, Kassner A. Evolution of blood-brain-barrier permeability after acute ischemic stroke. PLoS One. 2017;**12**(2):e0171558. DOI: 10.1371/journal.pone.0171558

[86] Da Fonseca ACC, Matias D, Garcia C, et al. The impact of microglial activation on blood-brain barrier in brain diseases. Frontiers in Cellular Neuroscience. 2014;**8**:362. DOI: 10.3389/fncel.2014.00362

[87] Liu L, Zhang X, Wang L, Yang R, Cui L, Li M, Du W, Wang S. The neuroprotective effects of Tanshinone IIA are associated with induced nuclear translocation of TORC1 and upregulated expression of TORC1, pCREB and BDNF in the acute stage of ischemic stroke. Brain Research Bulletin. 2010;**82**(3-4):228-233. DOI: 10.1016/j.brainresbull.2010.04.005

[88] Liu S et al. Acute bioenergetic intervention or pharmacological preconditioning protects neuron against ischemic injury. Journal of Experimental Stroke and Translational Medicine. 2013a;**6**(1):997-1003. Available at: http://ovidsp.ovid.com/ovidweb.cgi?T=JS&PAGE=reference&D=emed11&NEWS=N&AN=2013503321

[89] Gaudin A, Yemisci M, Eroglu H, Lepetre-Mouelhi S, Turkoglu OF, Dönmez-Demir B, Caban S, Sargon MF, Garcia-Argote S, Pieters G, Loreau O, Rousseau B, Tagit O, Hildebrandt N, Le Dantec Y, Mougin J, Valetti S, Chacun H, Nicolas V, Desmaële D, Andrieux K, Capan Y, Dalkara T, Couvreur P. Squalenoyl adenosine nanoparticles provide neuroprotection after stroke and spinal cord injury. Nature Nanotechnology. 2014; **9**(12):1054-1062. DOI: 10.1038/nnano.2014.274

[90] Alzheimer's Association. 2015 Alzheimer's disease facts and figures. Alzheimer's & Dementia: The Journal of the Alzheimer's Association. 2015;**11**(3):332-384. Available at: http://www.ncbi.nlm.nih.gov/pubmed/25984581

[91] Krstic D, Knuesel I. Deciphering the mechanism underlying late-onset Alzheimer disease. Nature Reviews Neurology. 2012;**9**(1):25-34. Available at: http://www.ncbi.nlm.nih.gov/pubmed/23183882

[92] Wu L et al. Early-onset familial Alzheimer's disease (EOFAD). The Canadian Journal of Neurological Sciences. Le journal canadien des sciences neurologiques. 2012;**39**(4):436-445. Available at: http://www.ncbi.nlm.nih.gov/pubmed/22728850 [Accessed December 8, 2016]

[93] Thompson SM. Neuroscience: Matching at the synapse. Science. 2005;**308**(5723):800-801

[94] Rodriguez-Vieitez E et al. Diverging longitudinal changes in astrocytosis and amyloid PET in autosomal dominant Alzheimer's disease. Brain. 2016;**139**(3):922-936

[95] Friedrich RP et al. Mechanism of amyloid plaque formation suggests an intracellular basis of Abeta pathogenicity. Proceedings of the National Academy of Sciences of the United States of America. 2010;**107**(5):1942-1947. Available at: http://www.pnas.org/content/107/5/1942.full

[96] Erickson MA, Banks WA. Blood-brain barrier dysfunction as a cause and consequence of Alzheimer's disease. Journal of Cerebral Blood Flow and Metabolism. 2013;**33**(10):1500-1513. DOI: 10.1038/jcbfm.2013.135

[97] Hardy J. The amyloid hypothesis for Alzheimer's disease: A critical reappraisal. Journal of Neurochemistry. 2009;**110**(4):1129-1134. DOI: 10.1111/j.1471-4159.2009.06181.x

[98] Kawarabayashi T, Younkin LH, Saido TC, Shoji M, Ashe KH, Younkin SG. Age-dependent changes in brain, CSF, and plasma amyloid (beta) protein in the Tg2576 transgenic mouse model of Alzheimer's disease. The Journal of Neuroscience. 2001;**21**(2):372-381

[99] Matsubara E, Ghiso J, Frangione B, Amari M, Tomidokoro Y, Ikeda Y, Harigaya Y, Okamoto K, Shoji M. Lipoprotein-free amyloidogenic peptides in plasma are elevated in patients with sporadic Alzheimer's disease and Down's syndrome. Annals of Neurology. 1999;**45**(4):537-541

[100] Iadecola C, Zhang F, Niwa K, Eckman C, Turner SK, Fischer E, Younkin S, Borchelt DR, Hsiao KK, Carlson GA. SOD1 rescues cerebral endothelial dysfunction in mice overexpressing amyloid precursor protein. Nature Neuroscience. 1999;**2**(2):157-161

[101] Blair LJ, Frauen HD, Zhang B, Nordhues BA, Bijan S, Lin YC, Zamudio F, Hernandez LD, Sabbagh JJ, Selenica ML, Dickey CA. Tau depletion prevents progressive blood-brain barrier damage in a mouse model of tauopathy. Acta Neuropathologica Commu nications. 2015;**3**:8. DOI: 10.1186/s40478-015-0186-2

[102] Liu Z, Gao X, Kang T, Jiang M, Miao D, Gu G, Hu Q, Song Q, Yao L, Tu Y, Chen H, Jiang X, Chen J. B6 peptide-modified PEG-PLA nanoparticles for enhanced brain delivery of neuroprotective peptide. Bioconjugate Chemistry. 2013b;**24**(6):997-1007. DOI: 10.1021/bc400055h

[103] Kurakhmaeva KB, Djindjikhashvili IA, Petrov VE, Balabanyan VU, Voronina TA, Trofimov SS, Kreuter J, Gelperina S, Begley D, Alyautdin RN. Brain targeting of nerve growth factor using poly(butyl cyanoacrylate) nanoparticles. Journal of Drug Targeting. 2009 Sep;**17**(8):564-574. DOI: 10.1080/10611860903112842

[104] Wang ZH, Wang ZY, Sun CS, Wang CY, Jiang TY, Wang SL. Trimethylated chitosan-conjugated PLGA nanoparticles for the delivery of drugs to the brain. Biomaterials. 2010;**31**(5):908-915. DOI: 10.1016/j.biomaterials.2009.09.104

[105] Titova N, Padmakumar C, Lewis SJG, Chaudhuri KR. Parkinson's: A syndrome rather than a disease? Journal of Neural Transm (Vienna). Aug 2017;**124**(8):907-914. DOI: 10.1007/s00702-016-1667-6. Review [Epub 2016 Dec 27]. PubMed PMID: 28028643; PubMed Central. PMCID: PMC5514217.

[106] Pisani V, Stefani A, Pierantozzi M, et al. Increased blood-cerebrospinal fluid transfer of albumin in advanced Parkinson's disease. Journal of Neuroinflammation. 2012;**9**:188. DOI: 10.1186/1742-2094-9-188

[107] Kortekaas R, Leenders KL, van Oostrom JC, Vaalburg W, Bart J, Willemsen AT, et al. Blood-brain barrier dysfunction in parkinsonian midbrain in vivo. Annals of Neurology. 2005;**57**:176-179. DOI: 10.1002/ana.20369

[108] Gray MT, Woulfe JM. Striatal blood-brain barrier permeability in Parkinson's disease. Journal of Cerebral Blood Flow and Metabolism. 2015;**35**(5):747-750. DOI: 10.1038/jcbfm.2015.32

[109] Barcia C, Bautista V, Sánchez-Bahillo A, Fernández-Villalba E, Faucheux B, Poza y Poza M, Fernandez Barreiro A, Hirsch EC, Herrero MT. Changes in vascularization in substantia nigra pars compacta of monkeys rendered parkinsonian. Journal of Neural Transmission (Vienna). 2005;**112**(9):1237-1248

[110] Rite I, Machado A, Cano J, Venero JL. Blood-brain barrier disruption induces in vivo degeneration of nigral dopaminergic neurons. Journal of Neurochemistry. 2007;**101**(6): 1567-1582

[111] Bartels AL. Blood-brain barrier P-glycoprotein function in neurodegenerative disease. Current Pharmaceutical Design. 2011;**17**(26):2771-2777 Review

[112] Leveugle B, Faucheux BA, Bouras C, Nillesse N, Spik G, Hirsch EC, Agid Y, Hof PR. Cellular distribution of the iron-binding protein lactotransferrin in the mesencephalon of Parkinson's disease cases. Acta Neuropathologica. 1996;**91**(6):566-572

[113] Huang R, Han L, Li J, Ren F, Ke W, Jiang C, Pei Y. Neuroprotection in a 6-hydroxydopamine-lesioned Parkinson model using lactoferrin-modified nanoparticles. The Journal of Gene Medicine. 2009;**11**(9):754-763. DOI: 10.1002/jgm.1361. PubMed PMID: 19554623

[114] Hu K et al. Lactoferrin-conjugated PEG–PLA nanoparticles with improved brain delivery: In vitro and in vivo evaluations. Journal of Controlled Release. 2011;**134**(1):55-61. Available at: http://www.ncbi.nlm.nih.gov/pubmed/19038299 [Accessed January 19, 2017]

[115] Duncan R, Gaspar R. Nanomedicine(s) under the microscope. Molecular Pharmaceutics. 2011;**8**(6):2101-2141. Available at: http://www.ncbi.nlm.nih.gov/pubmed/21974749

[116] Wang AZ, Langer R, Farokhzad OC. Nanoparticle delivery of cancer drugs. Annual Review of Medicine. 2012;**63**:185-198. Available at: http://www.ncbi.nlm.nih.gov/pubmed/21888516

[117] Howard MD et al. PEGylation of nanocarrier drug delivery systems: State of the art. Journal of Biomedical Nanotechnology. 2008;**4**(2):133-148

[118] Nicolas J et al. Design, functionalization strategies and biomedical applications of targeted biodegradable/biocompatible polymer-based nanocarriers for drug delivery. Chemical Society Reviews. 2013;**42**(3):1147-1235. Available at: http://www.ncbi.nlm.nih.gov/pubmed/23238558

[119] Corot C et al. Recent advances in iron oxide nanocrystal technology for medical imaging. Advanced Drug Delivery Reviews. 2006;**58**(14):1471-1504

[120] Jain KK. Nanobiotechnology-based strategies for crossing the blood–brain barrier. Nanomedicine. 2012;**7**(8):1225-1233. Available at: http://www.futuremedicine.com/doi/abs/10.2217/nnm.12.86

[121] Lesniak MS, Brem H. Targeted therapy for brain tumours. Nature Reviews Drug Discovery. 2004;**3**(6):499-508. Available at: http://www.nature.com/doifinder/10.1038/nrd1414

[122] Abbott NJ, Rönnbäck L, Hansson E. Astrocyte–endothelial interactions at the blood–brain barrier. Nature Reviews Neuroscience. 2006;**7**(1):41-53. Available at: http://www.nature.com/doifinder/10.1038/nrn1824

[123] Vlieghe P, Khrestchatisky M. Medicinal chemistry based approaches and nanotechnology-based systems to improve CNS drug targeting and delivery. Medicinal Research Reviews. 2013;**33**(3):457-516 Available at: http://doi.wiley.com/10.1002/med.21252

[124] Agulla J et al. In Vivo Theranostics at the Peri-infarct region in cerebral ischemia. Theranostics. 2014;**4**(1):90-105. Available at: http://www.thno.org/v04p0090.htm

[125] Asahi M et al. Antiactin-targeted immunoliposomes ameliorate tissue plasminogen activator-induced hemorrhage after focal embolic stroke. Journal of Cerebral Blood Flow & Metabolism. 2003;**23**(8):895-899. Available at: http://gateway.ovid.com/ovidweb.cgi?T=JS&PAGE=crossref&AN=00004647-200308000-00002

[126] Bana L et al. Liposomes bi-functionalized with phosphatidic acid and an ApoE-derived peptide affect Aβ aggregation features and cross the blood–brain-barrier: Implications for therapy of Alzheimer disease. Nanomedicine: Nanotechnology, Biology and Medi cine. 2014;**10**(7):1583-1590. Available at: http://linkinghub.elsevier.com/retrieve/pii/S1549963413006849

[127] Costa PM et al. MiRNA-21 silencing mediated by tumor-targeted nanoparticles combined with sunitinib: A new multimodal gene therapy approach for glioblastoma. Journal of Controlled Release: Official Journal of the Controlled Release Society. 2015;**207**:31-39. Available at: http://www.ncbi.nlm.nih.gov/pubmed/25861727 [Accessed September 23, 2015]

[128] Deddens LH et al. MRI of ICAM-1 upregulation after stroke: The importance of choosing the appropriate target-specific particulate contrast agent. Molecular Imaging and Biology. 2013;**15**(4):411-422

[129] Karathanasis E et al. MRI mediated, non-invasive tracking of intratumoral distribution of nanocarriers in rat glioma. Nanotechnology. 2008;**19**(31):315101. Available at: http://www.ncbi.nlm.nih.gov/pubmed/21828778\ [Accessed August 19, 2015]

[130] Li XT et al. Multifunctional targeting daunorubicin plus quinacrine liposomes, modified by wheat germ agglutinin and tamoxifen, for treating brain glioma and glioma stem cells. Oncotarget. 2014;**5**(15):6497-6511. Available at: http://www.ncbi.nlm.nih.gov/pubmed/25153726

[131] Liu Y et al. Brain-targeted co-delivery of therapeutic gene and peptide by multifunctional nanoparticles in Alzheimer's disease mice. Biomaterials. 2016;**80**:33-45

[132] Liu Y et al. Multifunctional tandem peptide modified paclitaxel-loaded liposomes for the treatment of vasculogenic mimicry and cancer stem cells in malignant glioma. ACS Applied Materials & Interfaces. 2015;**7**(30):16792-16801. Available at: http://pubs.acs.org/doi/abs/10.1021/acsami.5b04596

[133] Mohamed MS et al. Structurally distinct hybrid polymer/lipid nanoconstructs harboring a type-I ribotoxin as cellular imaging and glioblastoma-directed therapeutic vectors. Macromolecular Bioscience. 2014;**14**(12):1696-1711

[134] Peiris PM et al. Treatment of invasive brain tumors using a chain-like nanoparticle. Cancer Research. 2015;**75**(7):1356-1365. Available at: http://cancerres.aacrjournals.org/content/early/2015/01/27/0008-5472.CAN-14-1540.abstract

[135] Rotman M et al. Enhanced glutathione PEGylated liposomal brain delivery of an anti-amyloid single domain antibody fragment in a mouse model for Alzheimer's disease. Journal of Controlled Release. 2015;**203**:40-50. Available at: http://linkinghub.elsevier.com/retrieve/pii/S0168365915001121

[136] Wang L et al. Co-delivery of 5-fluorocytosine and cytosine deaminase into glioma cells mediated by an intracellular environment-responsive nanovesicle. Polymer Chemistry. 2014;**5**(15):4542-4552. Available at: http://xlink.rsc.org/?DOI=C4PY00291A

[137] Xia C-F et al. Intravenous glial-derived neurotrophic factor gene therapy of experimental Parkinson's disease with Trojan horse liposomes and a tyrosine hydroxylase promoter. The Journal of Gene Medicine. 2008;**10**(3):306-315. Available at: http://doi.wiley.com/10.1002/jgm.1152

[138] Xiang Y et al. Chlorotoxin-modified stealth liposomes encapsulating levodopa for the targeting delivery against the Parkinson's disease in the MPTP-induced mice model. Journal of Drug Targeting. 2012;**20**(1):67-75. Available at: http://www.tandfonline.com/doi/full/10.3109/1061186X.2011.595490

[139] Yang ZZ et al. Enhanced brain distribution and pharmacodynamics of rivastigmine by liposomes following intranasal administration. International Journal of Pharmaceutics. 2013;**452**(1-2):344-354. Available at: http://dx.doi.org/10.1016/j.ijpharm.2013.05.009